UNDERSTANDING RESEARCH

UNDERSTANDING RESEARCH

RESEARCH

a scientific approach for health care professionals

PAUL STEVENS
ANNETTE SCHADE
BARRY CHALK
OLIVER SLEVIN

British Library Cataloguing-in-Publication Data

Stevens, P.J.M.
    Understanding research : a scientific approach for
    health care professionals.
    I. Title II. Schade, A.L. III. Chalk, B. IV. Slevin, O. D'A.
    610.73072

    ISBN 1-873732-02-3

Cover design:
Artisan Graphics, Edinburgh.

Typeset in 10/12 Palatino
by Word Power, Berwickshire.

Translated sections by
L.F.M. van Beeck

Printed and bound by
The Alden Press, Oxford.

© 1993 Campion Press Limited
384 Lanark Road,
Edinburgh EH13 0LX

The extracts on pages 17, 18, 24, 27-32, 59, 61, 62, 77, 93, 94 are taken from articles in
Nursing Research, British Medical Journal and *Journal of Advanced Nursing.*

THE AUTHORS

Oliver Slevin is Chief Executive Officer at the National Board for Nursing, Midwifery and Health Visiting in Northern Ireland. He previously occupied clinical and teaching posts in Northern Ireland, Scotland and England. Dr. Slevin's particular interest in the role of research in the Project 2000 curriculum is reflected in this book.

Barry Chalk gained experience as a qualified nurse for some years before being appointed as a course tutor with responsibilities for general nursing students and an Enrolled Nurse (Mental) programme. There followed education management posts and at present he is Vice Principal at Newcastle and Northumbria College of Health.

Annette Schade studied Educational Psychology at the State University in Groningen where she specialised in Clinical Psychology and Medical Sociology. She now lectures in Psychology and Sociology at a college of higher education in the Netherlands.

Paul Stevens is an experienced nurse in various fields of health care including management and nursing home care. At present he is a lecturer at a college of higher education in the Netherlands. His particular areas of interest are Innovation, Counselling and Information Technology in Education.

GUEST CONTRIBUTOR

Kader Parahoo is a senior lecturer in the Department of Nursing at the University of Ulster. He has been teaching Nursing Research to undergraduates and postgraduates for a number of years. Dr. Parahoo has carried out research on community psychiatric nursing and clinical teaching. He has also written a number of articles on nursing research. His main clinical interest is in the field of psychiatric nursing. Dr Parahoo wrote Chapter 11 and jointly wrote Chapters 3 and 5 with Dr. Slevin.

INTRODUCTION

Interest in scientific research within the caring professions appears to be growing at an ever increasing pace.

This may partly be explained by the desire of the professions to meet the needs and demands of their consumers, the patients and clients. Of equal importance however is a shift in the objectives of vocational education. Developments in both the subject areas and the professions are occurring so quickly that education is scarcely able to keep pace and incorporate the changes formally in the curriculum. It is necessary therefore that more attention is paid to the primary skills which help students to follow these developments, so that they may familiarise themselves with the advances whenever necessary and be able to apply them in professional practice. Insight into the outcomes of scientific research and the ability to critically evaluate research studies and reports is one of these skills.

In looking more specifically at the nursing profession, a number of reasons can be found for the growing interest in research:

 – At a *macro level*, that of *professional practice*, it can be seen that the scientific development of nursing stimulates an increase in professionalism amongst nurses. The converse is equally true, that professionalism encourages interest in research.

 – At the *level of collective professional practice*, more and more nurses are encouraged and required to put the results of research into practice or give stimulus to and make suggestions for research based upon their practical experience.

 – At the *level of individual professional practice*, the *micro level*, nurses should increasingly be able to account for their actions in terms of knowledge which has been scientifically verified. Insight into research can also be helpful in studying literature and reports and in making personal notes. During educational programmes or courses this insight will support course work, for instance in the writing of assignments and study activities.

This book is intended to contribute toward the understanding of research for nurses, students of nursing and the professions allied to medicine, thus making a contribution to the further development of these professions. It is not our intention that after studying this text the readers will be capable of developing and carrying out research on their own. A deeper study of the subject material will be required to achieve that standard. Its aim, therefore, is to provide students of nursing and the paramedical professions with insight into the process of research.

This general aim will be achieved by familiarising readers with and giving them insight into:
- the significance of scientific research for professional practice;
- the process of developing scientific theory and the importance of empirical research;
- the research cycle, its phases and their interdependence;
- the variety of research designs, different research strategies and their use;
- current statistical concepts, particularly of descriptive statistics;
- the development of skills for assessing and interpreting research reports.

In relation to the structure and use of the book a number of points should be noted by the reader. The introductory chapter deals with the concept of science in general and then focuses on science related to nursing and professions allied to medicine. In Chapter Two the research process in general is described. This chapter addresses the research process from a predominantly positivistic and mainly quantitative perspective. Chapter Three concentrates on the qualitative perspective which is an important approach adopted in some social scientific and health care orientated research. Chapters Four to Ten each deal with a major stage in the research process. In Chapter Eleven the importance of the ability to critically evaluate a research project is emphasised and the skills necessary to this important activity are addressed. Chapter Twelve, the concluding chapter, considers the importance of research in the caring professions and in particular looks to future developments in care-orientated research. To assist understanding and assimilation of the information provided, examples and study activities are given.

The authors would welcome any constructive observations or suggestions which contribute to the objective of this book, the publication of which was made possible through the direct and indirect support of others. They would like to thank all those people involved.

Spring 1993
Paul Stevens
Annette Schade
Barry Chalk
Oliver Slevin

CONTENTS

1

THE SCIENTIFIC PERSPECTIVE

1.1 INTRODUCTION: A DEFINITION

There are diverse and often stereotyped ideas about science and the scientist. The absent-minded professor, a dusty, scholarly person preoccupied with important matters of which the common man is ignorant, working long hours in an ivory tower — this is one popular image of the scientist.

It is not our intention to discuss stereotyped notions of science in this chapter, but rather to put forward a more realistic view of science.

'Science' may be defined as 'a coherent system of knowledge about the world (or a part of it)'.

1.1.1 *Science as an outcome*

In this concept there is a strong emphasis on knowledge, the body of knowledge which science has built up about the world. However, consideration must be given to what this knowledge consists of and how it is structured. (These are in effect cognitive questions on issues of epistemological, that is, issues of the nature and structure of knowledge.) Connected with this is the question of establishing truth within the acquired knowledge and the problem of conceptua-lising that knowledge and its meanings.

1.1.2 *Science as an activity*

Science can also be defined in terms of 'scientific pursuit' or 'research'.
The questions here are about how science or research builds up knowledge and which methods are at the scientist's disposal to acquire this knowledge. This is *Science as an activity*. In this respect methodological problems are posed, involving questions about the problem of perception. Where research is anchored in the perception of reality, the question emerges as to how pure and unbiased human perception can be.
A second question touches upon the problem of induction (i.e. reasoning which draws general conclusions from specific instances). How far can a universal state-ment be justified on the basis of a large number of observations? The problem area here is one of verification or falsification. This problem can be illustrated with the example of the black and white ravens.
Research carried out on the colour of ravens discovers after repeated examination in a variety of locations that ravens are black. The question which then arises is:
> 'Can it be concluded that all ravens are black, despite the fact that not every raven which exists has been examined?'

Verification of this statement will be confirmed partially but increasingly by ongoing examination of the colour of ravens. From the point of view of falsification the statement can be accepted as true until disproved. It will be clear that both verification and falsification address the inductive problem, but from different perspectives.

A third problem relates to theoretical conceptualisation; how do scientists arrive at theoretical concepts according to which verifiable scientific questions can be formulated?

STUDY ACTIVITY 1
Give a more extensive explanation of the term *induction*. Use the following examples:
a. cars as four-wheeled vehicles
b. cats as animals with tails.

1.1.3 Formal and empirical sciences
Before moving on further to define the various concepts, the term 'science' should itself be examined. Wherever reference in this book is made to science and the pursuit of scientific studies, the empirical sciences are meant, and not the formal sciences. The *formal* sciences focus on the roles and quality of reasoning (as, for instance, in the cases of mathematics, logic and philosophy). The *empirical* sciences on the other hand focus on what we can learn through interaction with the real world.

1.2 OBJECTIVES OF SCIENCE

1.2.1 The search for knowledge
There are many motives for the pursuit of science. The eagerness to solve everyday problems and curiosity about the world in which humans exist have always been important. In present-day western society the objectives of science can be described as:
    a. the formulation of *explanatory* theories concerning empirical reality and the testing of these theories against reality. Scientists try to comprehend the world and to explain the phenomena which occur in this world;
    b. the development of solutions to practical problems.

These objectives can be looked upon as two extremes of a continuum. The first concentrates on knowledge for the sake of knowledge without that knowledge having any immediate application. The second focuses on the practical application of scientific insights. In this instance applicability is a priority.
This distinction defines the difference between fundamental (also known as pure scientific, theory-orientated or explanatory) research and practical (also known as applied, policy-orientated or action-orientated) research.

1.2.2 Fundamental or pure research and applied research

Fundamental research is directed at generating knowledge for its own sake. The creation of scientific theory has first priority. The direct usefulness of the results of fundamental research is limited, certainly in the short term.

> An example of this might be research into whether the onset of psychological problems associated with ageing can be described as 'adaptation', helping to preserve 'health' through adjustment to a changing physical, social and cultural environment. Such an investigation might reinforce the validity of the adaptation theory in relation to the preservation of health and the onset of disease.

Applied research, however, is triggered by a practical question or problem, with the results of the research being capable of immediate use.

> An investigation by a Health Authority into the effect of different working patterns of district nurses on the quality of preventive care for the elderly, could be an example of applied research.

Yet the contrast is not as great or as clear-cut as is suggested here. Much applied research uses theories which have been devised as a result of fundamental research to solve the problems presented. And, conversely, applied research can provide an important incentive for the formation or revision of theories. Thus the following could happen in relation to the examples mentioned above:

– starting from a growing confirmation of the adaptation theory to explain the occurrence of disease, applied research might be undertaken to assess the impact of living conditions on the occurrence of illness among the elderly. On this basis political and social decisions might be taken;

– research indicates that a variety of tasks have a positive effect on the quality of care. This could stimulate a further theoretical investigation to discover which factors in, say, the 'human resources' organisation theories are linked with differentiated tasks. Examining the theoretical principles which account for this positive effect would test the 'human resources' theory and might further corroborate it.

STUDY ACTIVITY 2

Indicate whether the following questions are examples of pure or applied research, or whether they can be fitted into both kinds of research.

a. What is the impact of socio-economic status and lifestyle on the health of five and six year olds?

b. Is there less truancy at schools with a more traditional style of education than at schools with a more progressive or innovative style?

c. In what way are self-reliance and social support related in the case of a person with rheumatoid arthritis living at home?

d. What is the effect of artificial lighting on restlessness among elderly people?

e. What are the effects on teaching results of organising a training programme according to subjects as compared to organising one according to themes?

1.3 PREMISES AND GUIDING PRINCIPLES OF RESEARCH

1.3.1 Points of departure

In seeking explanatory theories concerning empirical reality, the researcher is guided by a number of aims:

— *Enhancing human rationality and stripping it of myths and superstition by searching for truth.* Within this concept truth means 'agreement with the facts' and hence this is a relative notion of truth and not an absolute one of, 'that is how it is, and it will always remain so'...

— A second important aim is *to achieve maximum information*. The greater our knowledge becomes, the more uncomprehended situations will be demystified. This implies that science does not, as a rule, seek social acceptance. Orthodoxy (socially accepted 'truth') has been debunked by the results of research more than once. Think for example of earlier beliefs that the world was flat, or that the sun revolves around the earth.

— *Striving for simplicity* constitutes a third objective of research. As a general rule it can be stated that simple theories are more expressive than complex theories.

— *Seeking after valid knowledge,* the fourth aim, implies that deductions should be logically structured and the chosen line of argument should be built up correctly.

— *The findings of research should have utility.* This fifth aim does not mean that the findings of research should be purely practice-orientated. It does mean, however, that they should be valid for a specific situation.

The above objectives are shared by the majority of researchers. In addition there are a number of premises which are more controversial, like the pursuit of efficiency, freedom from social value judgements, and the emancipatory character of scientific work.

> As an illustration of this consider the development of the atomic bomb. Can the scientists who made the bomb argue that they acted exclusively from scientific motives and that the consequences of this invention are a political and social affair and are not part of scientific work?

Scientific knowledge leads to a certain control of and influence on reality. Frequently, the exercise of this control and influence gives rise to heated discussion.

STUDY ACTIVITY 3

Contemporary genetic technology makes it possible to identify those couples who have a high probability of producing children with serious deformities. Which minimum conditions should be met, in your view, before these techniques may be further developed and applied?

It should be emphasised here that research and scientific studies do not exclude value judgment and sincere personal interest, particularly where the choice of subjects and the personal standpoint of the scientists are concerned. Science as such, however, attempts to be value-free and pure, focusing exclusively on objective truth. Indeed, the enormous growth of research and its results have fostered the idea that scientific explanations and solutions are available for all issues. Account should also be taken of the increasing involvement of scientists in current affairs programmes on television and in the other media, where they often make a substantial contribution to discussions which are subjective rather than scientific.

It would be very naive to say that scientists themselves are not partially responsible for any confusion about their role. They have regularly spoken freely, despite the fact that in essence questions of a subjective and personal nature are claimed to be outside the domain of science.

1.3.2 Research conditions

From the objectives and guiding principles described, a number of criteria may be deduced which the research process should meet. These are known as *methodological ground rules*. The term 'method' here is used in its original sense, viz... 'the way along which...'. In this case, it refers to the way along which knowledge is built up. Stemming from this the following *conditions* for scientific research will be reasonably self-evident.

– *Objectivity*. This means that research is not a personal affair, but ought to be of general validity and free from personal interpretation or subjective bias.

– Wherever objectivity is not possible, the aim is *intersubjective knowledge* (i.e. knowledge or data which is presented by more than one person, and preferably, by a great number of people, thus giving it the strength of general acceptance or inter-observer agreement).

– *Verifiability*. It should be clear how the investigation was carried out and how the results and conclusions were arrived at. Only then does criticism of the conclusions become possible and only then can the inquiry be refuted or verified.

– *Openness and accessibility* of the research method used and of the knowledge acquired are necessary to be able to meet the previous condition.

– The knowledge acquired should be built up *systematically* and unambiguously formulated. When there is confusion about what is meant, refutation or verification are not possible.

STUDY ACTIVITY 4

a. Study a chapter in a textbook devoted to the subject of 'wound care'. Check whether the knowledge described there meets the conditions mentioned above.
b. Carry out the same study activity for the following excerpt on the validity of different methods of measuring body temperature of post-operative patients. What differences do you encounter? What can you conclude on the basis of this?

Monitoring of body temperature in the postoperative period is an important nursing function. Selection of site and instrument is usually left to the individual nurse's discretion. Understanding of the relationships between site, instrument, and core body temperature is necessary for informed decision making.

The findings of this study suggest that for the postoperative patient the best reflection of core body temperature is a rectal temperature measurement, taken with a mercury thermometer for 5 minutes. It must be noted that on average this rectal temperature will be 0.5°C higher than core body temperature. The next best indicator of core body temperature is an axillary temperature measurement taken with a mercury thermometer for 10 minutes. This measurement will be slightly lower (0.2°C) than core body temperature. Axillary temperatures obtained with an electronic thermometer are the poorest reflection of core body temperature of the three methods tested. On average, axillary temperatures taken with an electronic thermometer are 0.6°C lower than core body temperature. This difference should be taken into consideration when instituting measures to rewarm awake, noncardiac postoperative patients who neither complain of coldness, nor shiver.

A finding of importance is the relation-ship between postoperative core body temperature and age. Earlier work notes that the elderly are susceptible to accidental hypothermia (Reuler, 1978). The correlation of −0.64 between age and postoperative core body tempera-ture suggests that the elderly are also susceptible to hypothermia in a surgical setting. This finding points out the ne-cessity of careful observation for post-operative hypothermia in the elderly. Additional research should be done to determine whether the elderly are at increased risk for the effects of tempera-ture on postoperative drug (anesthesia) excretion and other problems associ-ated with hypothermia in the post-operative period.

T. Heidenreich and M. Giuffre (1990), 'Postoperative temperature measurement', in: *Nursing Research* 39/3, pp. 153–154

1.3.3 The scientific forum

Safeguards for suitable research conditions are laid down in the *scientific forum*. This should not be conceived as a distant body handing down wisdom. Rather, it is fellow scientists who judge the scientific merit of research. The previously mentioned conditions function as points of departure. In addition, there are self-evident implicit standards and rules which should be obeyed. For example work must not be falsified, results must not be suppressed, and conditions which might cast a different light on the results obtained must not be concealed.

The verification by the scientific community, as described, usually takes place at the moment the results are published. Assessment for publication is a gauge for the scientific quality of the research. Some professional journals do publish when the research was methodologically less convincing, but nevertheless contained poten-tially interesting facts. Scientific journals make high demands before publication is considered. There is international recognition of journals of high scientific repute. Publication in renowned journals yields more respect than in less reputable ones. The *Journal of Advanced Nursing* for instance, has a solid reputation. Accordingly, articles in that journal will be verified by a broader scientific forum and will usually be of a higher scientific quality than articles in less prestigious journals.

Consultations with fellow scientists, e.g. at congresses and seminars, help to main-tain scientific standards. Researchers present research plans and the initial results of current projects. Constructive criticism from colleagues and the process of peer review both also contribute to the quality of the research.

Last but not least, critical verification takes place within academic institutions. Often separate research projects are part of a broader research study and so the quality of the individual project is of great importance to the others in that study. It is also often the case that other researchers attempt to replicate a piece of research, thus confirming or bringing into question its methods, data, findings etc. Replication is an important means by which the scientific community confirms the reliability and validity of knowledge.

1.4 THE CONVENTIONAL MODEL OF SCIENCE: THE EMPIRICAL CYCLE
Science can be regarded as an exact and rational activity, and it is possible to establish a model of the scientific process based on this view. The model, often called the standard model of present day science, is shown here in a simplified version.
The construction of the standard model should be regarded as:
  – an epistemological concept or model of science rather than a scientific process along which the actual research runs. This is discussed in Chapter 2 'The research process';
  – a simplified representation of science; science seen exclusively as a *rational* activity and not as a psychological, sociological or historical activity.

It is assumed that complete scientific theories exist in which all parts and their mutual connections are visible. This standard model is not yet recognisable as such in the case of a developing science such as 'nursing science'.

The empirical cycle, Figure 1.1, describes how theories are formed and justified in empirical science.

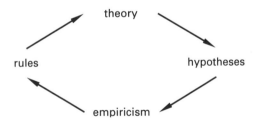

Figure 1.1 The empirical cycle

Explanation
All empirical knowledge emanates ultimately from perception. It is fundamental that this perceptual basis is independent of theory. This means that theories can be altered on the grounds of their perceptual basis, but that basis itself is not affected by the alteration of the theory. A fundamental criticism of this view is given later in this chapter.
On the strenth of data collected from the perceptual basis, empirical rules are arrived at through induction and generalisation. This inductive step should not be conceived as being static and self-evident; often generalisations are possible on the strength of the collected data. There is also a creative input. The rules, once established, offer the possibility of explaining phenomena. These rules are, like the perceptual basis, independent of theory. A change in the theoretical superstructure will not affect them.

Theories designed on the strength of the empirical basis ought to supply an explanation for the rules which have been invoked. The theory is a form of logical arrangement of empirical rules and a construction which provides a deeper insight into empirical reality. A theory describes an explanatory basis or underlying principle in accordance with which the rules occur.

An important condition attached to this theory therefore is that it allows us to predict or explain empirical patterns. A statement merely capable of explaining already-known rules is not referred to as a theory.

From the theory it should be possible to derive hypotheses which in their turn may be reduced to perceptible predictions. The hypothesis can be regarded as an anticipated empirical rule. A theory can be confirmed by verification of these new rules or hypotheses through empiricism or empirical investigation (research).

From this information, the question arises of whether current so-called theories in nursing or its allied professions can indeed be justified as theories; to what extent are they objective, based upon empirical rules, and capable of predictions?

1.5 CRITICISM OF THE STANDARD MODEL OF SCIENCE

In the standard model, science is conceived as an autonomous process, which starts from theory-dependent perceptual bases and is regulated by rational criteria. This standard model rests on two pillars: logic and empiricism, both described in the empirical cycle.

Factors of a socio-economic, political, cultural and personal nature are not relevant. They are not considered to have a potential impact. Fundamental criticism has been expressed of this standard model from various quarters. Two important critics are Karl Popper and Richard Kuhn:

1.5.1 Popper

Popper, a prominent British philosopher born in 1902, for the most part subscribed to the standard model. Yet he voiced fundamental criticism of a number of premises. First, he directs his criticism at the empirical basis of facts. He repudiates the idea of steady, independent perceptual bases, because an unbiased perceptual condition does not exist. In his view, supported by others, there is only theory-dependent perception. To put it simply, in perception humans use, often unconsciously, a set of concepts. This is why the same situation is perceived differently by different people. On the basis of this theory-dependent nature of perception, science, according to Popper (1963), should not focus on verifying or confirming this truth, but on refuting or falsifying it. This means that a theory in his view should be verifiable above all; the more a theory rules out the chance or random occurrence of phenomena, the more verifiable it is.

The more a theory can resist attempts at refutation, the stronger it is. Hence the concept of truth that Popper advocates is not based upon the best possible confirmation and agreement about the fact, but upon the falsification of untruth. The school that Popper represents is referred to as 'critical rationalism'.

1.5.2 Kuhn's paradigm concepts

Kuhn (1900-1967) provides a different outlook on scientific development. He looks at science from the perspective of world history and argues that the choice of certain concepts about science should ultimately be explained in psychological and socio-logical terms. He also contests the so-called gradual development of science; developments happen abruptly, as revolutions, instead of through evolution. Paramount in his theory is the concept of *'paradigm'* (Kuhn, 1962). A paradigm can be defined as a collection of postulates, laws, values and norms with respect to research, and a number of problem solutions.

In the so-called 'pre-paradigmatic' period of scientific discipline, the various theoretical views and trends contend with one another. There is no common basis and the discussion does not evolve beyond a debate over principles. The group of scientists which manages to solve concrete problems successfully on the basis of its principles wins the dispute. The principles will be largely influenced by social and psychological factors. A period of 'normal science' follows, when the paradigms and principles are determined by that group. The focus is on the strengthening of its paradigm.

During these periods of 'normal science' a number of matters, despite attempts at a solution, remain unsolved. When someone develops, often through a flash of insight, a different approach which not only allows for the explanation of the central problems but also helps to solve new ones, then this constitutes the new paradigm. Kuhn's ideas are controversial. His significance lies especially in the falsification of scientific rationality and the demonstration of the impact of internal and external factors on the development of science. He shows that any science is aiming at unification of its own paradigms and not at innovation or refutation of current theoretical views.

1.6 THE RELATIONSHIP OF RESEARCH TO PROFESSIONAL PRACTICE

How does research relate to professional practice? It could be asked to what extent researchers are able to support responsible professional practice with their knowledge? Conversely, it may be asked how far systematic professional practice can contribute to the accumulation of knowledge. The way in which science accumulates knowledge runs according to the pattern described in the empirical cycle. The way in which professionals do their jobs follows a course of methodological and system-atic action, such as *the systematic approach to care* (the nursing process). Both routes show significant similarities in their structures; the starting point of both processes is a definition of a problem. In both cases, this is followed by refinement of the questions and efforts at a solution by means of the systematic application of an appropriate conceptual tool-kit. The solution that is achieved is systematically evaluated in terms of the outcome.

In this sense, professional thinking is subject to the same discipline and is just as objective as scientific thinking. The professional, like the scientist, needs to reflect with sufficient detachment upon the situation and the actions to be taken. The motive for certain choices will have to be justified or verified and may prove contro-versial among colleagues. The justification of certain decisions within the concepts of a practice-theoretical framework corresponds to steps within the process of scientific study. The paradigms and theories of practice, based upon the reflections and developed traditions of problem solving, constitute a bridge between generalised scientific theories and individually-orientated thinking at the level of the concrete problem.

Generalised scientific theories also have a disciplinary function, offering theory and methodology which enhances responsible professionalism. In this way a contribution is made to practice.

There are also substantial differences between these activities:

    – their objectives are very different. Science looks for explanatory, predictive theories. The objective of practice is problem solving.

    – the reality that each concentrates on is also quite different. Science tries to arrive at general statements about a large area of reality, whereas practice attempts to arrive at concrete statements about specific situations.

    – practice therefore sets norms or prescribes standards. A desirable objective is pursued for the *specific* situation. Furthermore, professional practice inevitably enforces a normative attitude, whereas science basically takes freedom of value for granted, striving for pure statements.

    – the professional develops personal insights and conclusions based upon a sympathetic understanding and empathy, in combination with knowledge and experience. The scientist tends to take the 'hard' line of impersonal objectivitiy and statistical analysis.

The view endorsed by the authors is that there is a complementary relationship between scientists and professionals.

1.7 NURSING SCIENCE

1.7.1 The material object of nursing science
The material object of a science is based on the reality that one aims for. For example, the sick individual can be studied from various perspectives. The medical psychologist might look at the patient's sensations of pain, whereas the medical sociologist might consider the impact of the environment on the patient. In the case of nursing science, this material object is constituted by:

    – *processes and situations which require nursing*. Questions in this area include those related to the consequences of disease, handicap or treatment for the functioning of the patient. But the effects of health information on the functioning of the patient also come under this heading;

    – *the act of nursing*. This features elements such as nursing interventions and interactions between nurse and patient;

    – *the conditions of nursing*. This would include topics such as 'burn-out phenomena among nurses', 'the introduction of primary nursing', and 'quality differences between various forms of education and training for nurses';

    – *nursing in its social context*. Nursing must be considered as an integrated part of the social and health care system. Questions in this area concern the interaction between the social system and the phenomenon of nursing. International comparisons or historical studies can be classified under this heading.

1.7.2 The formal object of nursing and paramedical science

The formal object concerns the manner of studying empirical reality which is characteristic of the science. The medical psychologist and the medical sociologist, for example, have different methods as the two sciences adopt differing viewpoints. For each viewpoint there is a theoretical and conceptual framework and an individual research method which develops the reality for each science.

Nursing is still in its infancy as far as this is concerned. It is still establishing its own viewpoints and the accompanying research methodology. The result is that nursing continues to derive methods from other disciplines. Examples of conceptual models of nursing which are in use are the interaction model (Riehl, 1980), the adaptation model (Roy, 1980), and the self-care model (Orem, 1980).

It can therefore be said that, with respect to the formal object, there is still a preparadigmatic phase in nursing. The utility of theoretical models and visions are yet to be demonstrated. It does seem however that there is agreement about a kind of meta-paradigm. (This term refers to similarities between the various theories, characterised by the keywords 'man', 'environment', and 'health'.)

However, against the idea that nursing is in pre-paradigmatic phase, some argue that while the development of theories and models is presently in vogue, it should be regarded as only a phase in nursing. It is suggested that this phase has had little demonstrable effect on patient care as yet, that there is an absence of rational evidence showing that models work in practice and that the effects on professional practice are still unclear.

The conclusions drawn by the authors of this book are briefly that:
  – more attention should be given to multidimensional or pluralistic approaches using methods from various research traditions;
  – a similar pluralism concerning nursing theories should be used. Instead of a polarised approach between the various theoretical schools, co-operation involving the possible integration of different theories is suggested;
  – the fixed idea that the final result will be one all-explaining theory should be abandoned. Each construction and formulation of a theory ought to be viewed within the historical context of the evolution of theories;
  – a closer link between concrete professional practice and scientific studies should be established.

1.7.3 'Nursing research' or 'research in nursing'

The title of this section, 'nursing research' or 'research in nursing', represents a point of discussion which can be traced back to the material and formal objects of research. 'Nursing research' implies that research is done within the nursing domain (material object), by nurses, from a nursing point of view. This contrasts with, for example, the psychologist who researches the professional motivation of newly qualified nurses. While everything may appear clear conceptually and theoretically the formal object of nurses has scarcely been crystallised. As stated earlier, there is frequent borrowing from other sciences. Thus the discussion about whether there is 'nursing research' or 'research in nursing' is a recurrent theme.

STUDY ACTIVITY 5

Study the two summaries from the research articles below. Answer the following questions for each summary.

a. What is the material object of research?

b. What is the formal object of research?

c. Can you label it as 'nursing research' or 'research in nursing'?

1. This study was undertaken to determine the incidence and duration of diarrhea associated with tube feeding in critically ill adult patients who require mechanical ventilation. Of the 73 subjects studied, 63% had diarrhea associated with tube feeding. This incidence is higher than that reported from other studies of critically ill patients who were not mechanically ventilated. Multiple logistic regression analysis revealed that three variables (higher rates of infusion, greater tube-feeding osmolality, and change of tube-feeding product) were statistically significant predictors of diarrhea incidence. Antibiotic use and serum albumin levels were not predictors. In a stepwise multiple regression analysis, the duration of diarrhea was predicted by frequency of diarrhea, within the first 5 days of tube-feeding onset, tube-feeding product osmolality, and rate of tube-feeding infusion. Serum albumin levels and frequency of diarrhea beyond 6 days of tube-feeding onset did not predict duration of diarrhea. Higher osmolality and infusion rates of tube-feeding products did contribute to prediction of both incidence and duration of diarrhea.

C.E. Smith et al (1990), 'Diarrhea associated with tube feeding in mechanically ventilated critically ill patients', in: *Nursing Research* 39/3, pp. 148–152

2. One hundred nulliparous college female undergraduates were randomly assigned to a series of 10 treatment groups that comprised a variety of cognitive-behavioral pain-coping strategies designed as part of a labour preparation analogue. The efficacy of these treatments was subsequently assessed during a one-hour session involving twenty 80-sec exposures to a laboratory pain stimulus patterned to resemble labour contractions. Dependent variables included self-reported pain, systolic and diastolic blood pressure, frontalis EMG, and heart rate. One of the cognitive strategies – sensory transformation – was found to have a significant effect on self-reported pain. Analyses conducted on the other five dependent variables failed to show significant treatment effects.

E. Geden et al (1984), 'Self-report and psychophysiological effects of five pain-coping strategies', in: *Nursing Research* 33/5, pp. 260–265

1.7.4 *Importance of nursing research*

The significance of nursing research can be viewed from various levels of professional practice.

1. At the 'micro' level of professional practice the actions of the individual nurse are paramount. Nursing research expands knowledge of and insight into nursing problems and the nurse's actions. Research can contribute to the quality of direct nursing care and has an important function in helping to determine methodological

action, and in providing a scientifically based justification for professional choices.

2. At the 'meso' level of professional practice, the whole profession of nursing is the focus of attention. On this level, nursing research has a significant function relating to quality assurance and the maintenance of high professional standards. This can be achieved by the development of measuring techniques for the systematic assessment of quality.

3. The 'macro' level of professional practice concerns the function of the nursing profession in society. At this level nursing research must contribute to the structuring, underpinning and expansion of the domain of nursing knowledge and the professional practices which flow from it.

1.8 SUMMARY

This chapter focuses on the concept of 'science', firstly as an outcome and then, following some examples of epistemological problems, as an activity. A number of elementary methodological questions are also described.

The difference between formal and empirical sciences was then discussed. Subsequently, the focus moved to the objectives of science, explaining the differences and relationships between fundamental and applied research.

Following this introduction the premises and guiding principles of scientific pursuit were addressed. A description of the empirical cycle was given to represent the standard image of science. Criticism of this standard image was referred to. An analysis of the relationship between scientific studies concluded this general section.

The second part of the chapter focused on nursing science. Firstly attention was paid to the material and formal objects of this emergent scientific discipline, the formal object being subject to some discussion. Attention was also paid to the distinction between 'nursing research' and 'research in nursing' and the significance of such research to the nursing profession.

2

THE RESEARCH PROCESS

2.1 INTRODUCTION

In this chapter a general overview of the research process will be presented. This process starts with 'the issue' or problem and finishes with the writing of the research report.

It is possible to describe this process in a variety of ways. The different main phases can be presented in their component parts, or the process can be presented in general. The latter option is taken in this chapter. In later chapters each phase will be discussed in greater detail and dealt with more extensively.

Before proceeding it should be noted that the research process presented here is a model, and gives a more or less idealized representation of reality. Thus the 'nursing process' is a model for nursing practice. But models are not real – and, in reality, no single process will follow the ideal course.

In everyday research practice there will be ups and downs, and in some cases, fresh starts. The phases presented here in chronological order will not follow neatly, one after the other, each phase complete before the next is started. Some phases will occur concurrently. It is important therefore, when undertaking research, to continually anticipate possible intermediate modifications and amendments.

The following phases can be distinguished in the research process.

1. *The point of departure of the research.* Here the research issue or problem is identified. The issue or problem can arise from personal curiosity or scientific enthusiasm, it may have been raised by an employer, or by another external or internal stimulus;

2. *A review of the literature.* In order to provide the provisional inquiry with more background and greater depth, it is necessary to study the relevant literature about the problem area. It is possible that an answer to the question is already available;

3. *Making the issue operational.* This phase consists of setting the inquiry in motion after establishing its theoretical parameters. The central problem here is the correlation between the theoretical considerations and concepts and the practical execution of the research. Important stages here include: choosing an adequate research plan, involving the definition of a suitable statistical test, and developing reliable and valid yardsticks to measure the variables;

4. *The collection of data or data accumulation;*

5. *The processing and analysis of the data.* Raw data as the outcome of research, usually has little significance. Only after it has been analysed is it possible to draw conclusions;

6. *The research report.* The research processes and the results acquired are finally recorded in the research report. This report may for example be presented to an employer, be published, or constitute part of a further study.

2.2 THE PROBLEM

A research project starts off with a problem or question as point of departure. As was noted earlier, curiosity, theoretical involvement or some other stimulus (such as a final essay, exam paper or study activity) can be a point of departure for research.

Example
The rationale for an inquiry into the efficiency of a nursing course is:
– the rate of student drop-out from the course was investigated in an earlier inquiry which raised questions at the college; the impression existed, intuitively, that the actual wastage figures differed from the figures forecast for the college;
– staff at the college had been wondering for some time whether there might be a link between the successful completion of the nursing course and previous education. If it should become apparent that there is a link, then that would lead to modification of the admission policy.

A first question is usually not immediately suitable for research. Before it can be converted into a research topic, it is necessary to explore more deeply the problem area in which it is rooted. A theoretical frame of reference needs to be developed, as it were, for this first question. This exploration of the problem area is carried out through the study of the literature. A distinction needs to be made between *research literature* and *conceptual or theoretical literature*.

1. Research literature is about the factual research that has been carried out in the problem area concerned. It offers practical insight into earlier results of similar research, analysis techniques, measurement methods and the like. By studying the research literature the provisional question is focused and defined. It may even be answered on the basis of previous research results.

Example
In a research project on the comparision of rectal, axillary and sub-lingual temperatures in new-born infants, a summary of earlier research results can be found.

Torrance (1968) studied differences in simultaneous axillary and rectal temperature readings in 120 preterm infants. A mean difference of 0.05°C (0.09°F) was found between the sites when maximum temperature readings were compared. Torrance also reported that 95% of the subjects reached a stabilized axillary temperature in 4.5 minutes, whereas 90% reached stable rectal temperature in 3 minutes.

In a study of 30 full-term infants, Eoff, Meler and Miller (1974) compared simultaneous rectal and axillary readings. The mean difference of 0.49°F was statistically significant, although the clinical relevance of such a difference was questioned by the authors.

Schiffman (1982) took sequential axillary and rectal temperature readings in 46 full-term infants and found that, although all subjects reached stable rectal temperature in 5 minutes, only 63% of the subjects reached stable axillary temperature by 10 minutes. Comparison of the 10-minute rectal and axillary readings revealed a difference of 0.23°F.

Mayfield et al. (1984) studied axillary and

rectal temperature differences in 99 full-term and 44 preterm infants. Their findings of 0.59°F difference in full-term infants and 0.10°F difference in preterm infants supported the findings of Eoff et al. (1974) and Torrance (1968). However, the finding that 90% of both preterm and full-term subjects had stabilized temperatures by 5 minutes did not agree with Schiffman's (1982) findings.

Haddock, Vincent and Merrow (1986) compared sequential axillary and rectal readings in 30 full-term infants. Fifty-two percent of the subjects exhibited no difference between axillary and rectal readings, and an additional 42% had no more than a 0.4°F difference between readings. Mean difference between the two sites was 0.1°F, which did not support previous findings for full-term infants. The same investigators also found that 90% of the subjects reached optimum axillary temperature in 5 minutes, with the percentage of subjects rising to 94% in 10 minutes. All infants reached optimum rectal temperature in 4 minutes.

Moen, Chapman, Sheehan and Carter (1987) performed 12 sets of simultaneous axillary and rectal readings on each of 25 preterm infants. Comparisons of temperature differences at 3-, 5-, 8- and 10-minute readings revealed no more than 0.07°F difference between the two sites.

Stephan and Sexton (1987) studied increases in axillary temperatures in 60 full-term infants. Readings were taken at 90 seconds and 3, 5, 7 and 11 minutes. Temperatures in all infants continued to rise during the 11-minute period, and none reached stabilization.

Kunnel, O'Brien, Munro and Medoff-Cooper (1988) were the first to investigate the femoral/inguinal site as an alternative site for temperature monitoring. Simultaneous rectal, axillary, femoral and skin-to mattress temperatures were recorded each minute for 15 minutes in 99 full-term infants. Differences found between mean optimal temperatures were 0.09°F between axillary and inguinal sites, 0.35°F between rectal and inguinal sites and 0.26°F between rectal and axillary sites. Optimum placement times, which were defined as the time when 90% of subjects reach optimum temperature (Nichols, Ruskin, Glor & Kelly, 1966), were rectal, 5 minutes; axillary, 11 minutes; femoral, 11 minutes.

In their studies of preterm infants, Torrance (1968), Mayfield et al. (1984) and Moen et al. (1987) presented findings that support the supposition that this population has little difference between rectal and axillary temperature readings. In addition, there is agreement that preterm infants reach stable temperatures at both sites within 5 minutes.

In contrast, findings on full-term infant samples are not in agreement. Although Eoff et al. (1974) and Mayfield et al. (1984) found greater than a 0.49°F difference between rectal and axillary temperatures, Haddock et al. (1986), Kunnel et al. (1988) and Schiffman (1982), found less than 0.26°F difference between these sites. In addition, even though study findings by Eoff et al., Haddock et al. and Kunnel et al. agree that rectal temperature stabilization occurs within a 5-minute period, thermometer placement time for axillary temperature stabilization is not as clearly defined.

J. Bliss-Holtz (1989),
'Comparison of rectal, axillary and inguinal temperatures in full-term newborn infants',
in: *Nursing Research* 38/2, pp. 85-87

2. Conceptual literature, also called non-research literature, is especially intended to give greater insight into current theoretical concepts, thoughts and areas of disagreement. In addition the study of conceptual literature helps to make

theoretical concepts more concrete, and so improves understanding of the problem area.

Example

The following example concerns longitudinal research (an inquiry over a defined period of time, involving measurements at different stages) into factors precipitating the occurrence of stress among mothers and young children.

The 'stress' concept is, from a theoretical viewpoint, quite a challenge; what do we mean by stress and how do the researchers wish to use this concept in their research?

A brief example illustrates these considerations.

Theoretical Model of Stress: There are many theoretical views available for understanding stress and its effects on humans. Three major points of view alternatively depict stress as stimulus, response, and as interaction between person and environment (Cox, 1978; Derogatis, 1982). However, theoretical models of the stress process that integrate key components from among alternative views of stress are increasingly proposed (e.g. Pearlin, Menaghan, Lieberman & Mullan, 1981). In these, triggering events – often termed stressors – may define the beginning of a stress process. Appraisal or perception of stress, that is, judgment that an event is harmful or threatening to a person, mediates the responses to such events (Lazarus & Folkman, 1984). Social and personal resources may protect individuals or help them counterbalance the harmful effects of stress (Mercer, May, Ferketich & DeJoseph, 1986; Nuckolls, Cassel & Kaplan, 1972). Consequently, even though two individuals may experience a common stressor, they may not experience similar effects on health or parenting.

To better understand stress within the context of early parenting, Walker (1989) proposed a stress-process model that integrated findings from stress research with the concepts of role attainment and maternal identity (Mercer, 1981; Rubin, 1967a, 1967b, 1984). In that model, advent of a stressor initiates the stress process. Whether stressors exert adverse effects on the maternal role is mediated by mothers' perception or appraisal of stress. Because the maternal role is associated with imbalances between obligations and privileges (Baruch, Biener & Barnett, 1987), mothers' appraisals of stress may be manifested in general feelings of overload and unpredictability. It is the appraisal of stress that directly affects components of the maternal role, such as maternal identity and mothering behaviors. Additionally, mothers may actively engage in a health-promotive lifestyle (Walker, Sechrist & Pender, 1987) to manage or offset stress. A health-promotive lifestyle may act directly or as a buffer within the stress process, influencing either perception of stress or maternal role outcomes or both.

L.O. Walker (1989),
'A longitudinal analysis of stress process among mothers of infants',
in: *Nursing Research* 38/6, pp. 339-343

In many cases, however, the distinction between conceptual and research literature is not so easily made.

On the basis of a review of the literature the researcher can proceed to the definition of the final research question. This question requires clear formulation, and all of the concepts and elements in the question should be defined precisely.

It will also be clear from the above that the theoretical background and any other considerations related to the research question ought to have been clarified. This too usually follows on from the study of the literature.

In some research studies, there is a distinct conceptual model. Such a model consists of a coherent structure of concepts in which a theoretical vision of the problem is given and the connection between the various concepts is provided. From a coherent, theoretical base, it is possible to formulate clear expectations in advance. These are called *hypotheses* (see Chapter 4, section 4.3.4). The research then concentrates on the testing of these hypotheses.

2.3 CONVERTING THE RESEARCH PROBLEM INTO A RESEARCH SUBJECT

The research problem formulated in the first phase of the research process ought to be constructed in a way that facilitates further research in a specific situation.

The problem should be made measurable. Thus theoretical concepts will be translated into concrete activities related to actual persons or groups.

STUDY ACTIVITY 1

Analyse the article below in terms of the distinguishable phases of the research process. The research topic here is an investigation into disturbances of eating behaviour.

Research has been carried out on four wards. The patients can order their food a day and a half in advance. For dinner there is a choice from two main courses and three different sizes of portions, while a soup or dessert can be added.

The group
Three criteria were used for defining the research group: the patient should eat normally, be capable of answering questions and reside in a room where disturbances might occur. The (arbitrary) choice has been a room for at least three people, because in the case of fewer patients in a room the chance of disturbances becomes too small. In consultation with the ward sister it was decided which rooms would be involved in the experiment. The idea has been to collect data of patients over a period of five days at the most, because the turnover of patients made a longer study impossible. In the following sections the measuring methods used will be discussed briefly.

Food left over
A simple definition of food left-overs was: everything that the patient has left of the meal. Left-overs can be measured in different ways. For this experiment an objective measure has been used, the weight of the left-overs, and a subjective measure, the estimation of the left-overs of meat, vegetable or potatoes in relation to the order. This was possible because the order form, as part of the patient's tray, featured portion quantities. During the preparation, attempts were made to establish the initial weight but this method was too time-consuming, and the food cooled down.

Disturbance

The concept of 'disturbance' was defined as:

– the phenomenon of patients somehow being prevented from consuming their meal as they would wish to. In attempting to 'stimulate the appetite' and 'create a quiet atmosphere' anything which should be avoided has been called 'disturbance';

– an actual interruption of the meal when, for example, a doctor, visitor or fellow patient wants something from the patient;

– someone entering or leaving the room or presence of a third person, such as a nurse, a member of the domestic staff or a laboratory worker;

– change of the atmosphere which can be attributed to a fellow patient, for example, an inconvenient or unpleasant situation as a result of the fellow patient coughing up, vomiting or experiencing flatulence or diarrhoea.

The experiment will pay special attention to disturbances in the surroundings. The disturbances in the room are to be observed indirectly i.e. by recording persons walking in and out during the meal on a timed basis from the corridor. Participatory observation was not considered because of the 'disturbing' effect.

In general, three important phases of decision making can be distinguished in setting up an inquiry.

1. Which research plan (or design) is to be chosen? Thought needs to be given to the planning of various research steps and the controls that are to be established.

2. How are the concepts of the theoretical model used made measurable; which methods and techniques are applied in the collection of data; which existing instrument is chosen or which instruments should be developed?

3. In what way does random testing take place? Feasibility and target objectives play a part here.

2.3.1 The research design

The choice of a particular research plan is in fact strictly methodological, based on the connection between the theoretical concepts and the practical execution of the research. This connection should be clear and verifiable.

The following issues should be considered:

– how should certain results be interpreted later on?
– at what level will results be regarded as statistically significant?
– how might unexpected results be viewed?
– how many experimental and control groups are to be used?
– is there to be a measurement prior to or following the experiment?
– what sort of influence of variables is expected?.

Examples

1. In a piece of experimental research the usefulness of measuring techniques which can be used to evaluate proficiency training in health care is investigated. Groups composed of assorted participants are used to determine the effects of a range of variables (see the extract over).

31

To assess the background variables which might affect the test results, a questionnaire was presented to all participants during the experiment. Questions were asked about relevant training and work experience in health care. These data were particularly important because, for lack of *a priori* measurement, the initial level of the participants' experience was unknown.

Experimental Subjects

All practical work participants (16 persons) took part in the experiment. The practical placement constituted a first experience for them within a nursing environment. Because at the start of the practical experience the initial level of the participants' experience could not be determined, it was essential to include a number of persons whose initial characteristics would approximate to those of the participants in the practical placement. For this control group 13 first year undergraduate law students were selected at random. At the selection the condition had to be met that they had not undertaken any training or gained work experience in the nursing field. Owing to unforeseen circumstances, six participants of this control group did not participate in the experiment. A further 13 student nurses were asked to take part in the experiment to establish a level of reference (the reference group).

Research procedure

The participants were divided up into three random groups. Each group went through the experiment in a continuous sequence which lasted 160 minutes; 70 minutes for the proficiency test and 90 minutes for the other techniques. To avoid transfer of information between the test groups, the three groups were strictly separated thoughout the experiment. The observers did not know beforehand whether a participant belonged to the reference group, the control group or to the research group.

The observers were instructed beforehand in how to observe and score using a list of criteria. A co-observer simultaneously observed and scored the observers to assess their performances.

2. In a preliminary inquiry into job satisfaction amongst psychiatric nurses, the research procedure outlined in Figure 2.1 is found.

2.3.2 The method of data collection

In principle three main methods of data collection can be identified:
  – observation;
  – questioning;
  – measuring.

These different methods will be returned to in Chapter 7.

Study of the relevant literature will usually indicate which pre-existing instruments should be considered for use in the research. The employment of established instruments, or the development of one's own tools, will be indicated by the objectives of the research. For applied research, in a particular situation, the development of new instruments is more likely. With these, obscurities, uncertainties and

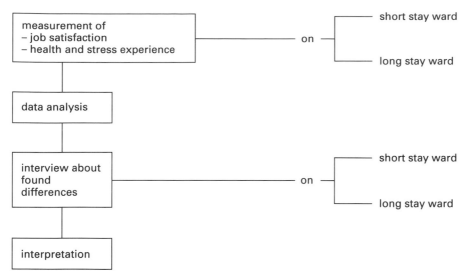

Figure 2.1 Research procedure for an inquiry into job satisfaction among psychiatric nurses.

problems regarding validity and reliability often arise. Reliability refers to constancy or consistency in whatever is measured. If a range of individuals carried out the same measurements in the same circumstances, the results should be the same. Simply put, validity means you measure only that which you wish to measure.

Data about validity and reliability are rarely available in the case of newly developed instruments. Such data will, however, be available in the case of those instruments and tools which have been tested before.

The concepts of reliability and validity will be returned to later.

2.3.3 The random sample

It is rarely possible for research to involve all the individuals to whom it will apply as only a part of that group or population is usually accessible to the researcher. A random sample is taken from this population. This should meet conditions of representativeness. The group which is invited to participate must be representative of the larger population from which it is drawn.

2.4 DATA COLLECTION

For this phase the general fixed rule applies that no alteration of the research design may be carried out once data collection has started. In this phase decisions taken earlier are put into practice.

Two aspects of this phase may be distinguished:
- the circumstances of data collection;
- the process of data collection.

2.4.1 The circumstances
- What form does the contact with respondents take? Is the communication oral or written, or both? The first can be very stimulating, but very time-consuming.

Sometimes it is possible to find an intermediate method where the researcher makes personal contact with a group of respondents, for example to explain the intentions of the study. The research is followed up and carried out in writing afterwards.

– What is the frequency of the contact? How often are data to be collected? For example, in an inquiry which tries to trace a certain development, how often will contact be made with the respondents (remembering that even a single meeting can be taxing for the respondents who may be children or who may be sick or elderly)?

– How will the respondents' confidentiality be protected? Is this carefully taken into account or hardly considered? The issue here is confidentiality during the course of the research and the impact of contact or confidentiality upon the process of data collection. In research reports the guarantee of confidentiality should be no problem, although the client who requested the research study can often be very curious about an individual respondent voicing a particular opinion.

– In which circumstances is the respondent required to function; individually or collectively? For example, in the case of data collection from group situations, observation techniques covering group interaction may be used.

– The practical aspects of the research come under this heading as well. As conducting research is a human activity, a few practical and administrative matters, such as telephone calls, appointments, memos, visits, etc. will have to be taken care of.

All of these questions which are related to the circumstances of the research should be answered from an academic perspective (from the point of view of the issue and the research plan) as well as on a practical level (what is efficient and effective).

2.4.2 *The process of data collection*

An important question under this heading is how respondents can be motivated to optimum levels of cooperation. One major factor is respect for the individuality and independence of the respondent. This respect and consideration should be made very apparent from the researcher's attitude towards keeping appointments, offering adequate explanations, and so on.

Secondly, it may be important to obtain the cooperation of key figures who may have some influence on the respondents. These may be people from the institutions and organisations which coordinate the research and who can encourage respondents to participate. Thirdly, clear explanation of the intention of the research and the giving of straightforward instructions may contribute to the motivation of the respondent. Finally the motivation of the researcher should be considered. If, for whatever reason, they do not appear interested or motivated, this attitude may be transferred to the respondents and key participants and affect responses.

It is often helpful as part of the process of data collection to record a diary of events. In this, the course of events during the research is laid down. It is thus possible to account retrospectively for events such as a respondent dropping out of the study. Another layer of insight can be based upon the experiences and opinions of respondents. These remarks might contribute to an explanation of the results or provide new stimuli to theory development. This can be significant especially in the case of qualitative research which seeks understanding and clarification in the creation of theoretical concepts.

Another very important question concerns the feasibility of the research plan and the handling of the tools to be employed. To this end it is important to carry out a pilot study, running through the research process on a small scale. Changes are still possible at this stage, before the research is carried out in its definitive form. As a general rule, however, it can be stated that during the actual data collection, alterations in the research plan and in the instruments used should no longer be made.

2.5 DATA ANALYSIS

Before data are collected, the researcher must have planned the analytical techniques which are to be used to analyse the information.

Because the raw material can be used more than once, it can be useful sometimes to apply different analytical techniques to meet specific purposes. Of course the researcher must be able to show how these choices fit within the total research plan. In the process of data analysis, at least two stages can be identified:

1. *The processing of data*. In the case of quantitative research large databases are often used which are encoded, making it necessary to have a listing of the codes together with the given values of the variables. The manual entering of data in a computer file is very labour intensive and can sometimes be assisted by the use of an optical character reader;

2. *The factual analysis*. For simple analyses (frequency distribution and determination of average, median, mode and dispersion) data are often more easily processed without a computer. This certainly applies when one is relatively unfamiliar with statistical programmes. For more complicated analyses a computer is indispensable.

Statistical methods (described more fully in Chapter 9)can be divided into two large groups: descriptive statistics and inferential statistics.

Some descriptive statistics are:

– analyses which confine themselves to one variable only, such as frequency distribution, average, dispersion etc.

– an analysis which refers to the relation between two variables such as the matrix and the correlation calculation

– analyses which involve more than two variables which affect each other simultaneously.

Inferential statistical methods, as the name suggests, are often applied for experimental and descriptive research. Of these, the variance-analysis and the t-test are commonly used.

2.6 REPORTING

This is the final phase in the research process. However this does not mean that the outcome of the literature study or the results of a pilot study are only written up now. These phases should naturally be completed earlier. The objective of reporting in a research paper is twofold:

- justification of the method adopted and the steps chosen.
- presentation of the results of the experiment, in the light of the framing of the problem.

Depending on the nature of the experiment, the report should contain a number of recommendations. These recommendations can relate to the actions to be undertaken, in the case of practical research, or to theoretical considerations in a fundamental experiment.

As far as layout is concerned, the research account should meet the general conditions for written reports. To present the research as well as possible, the following should receive particular attention:
- title, and subtitle if any;
- author(s);
- summary, or abstract;
- the context for the experiment;
- the formulated question or issue;
- its theoretical basis;
- the methodological approach identifying at least:
  - type of research and research design;
  - the sample;
  - instruments used;
- data analysis;
- results;
- conclusions, recommendations, points of discussion;
- bibliography or list of references cited.

2.7 SUMMARY

In this chapter research has been described in phases. Research can be triggered by an unanticipated occurrence, personal study or questions from clients. The research commences with a general issue. After a review of the literature this issue is specified. A precise indication is then given of what is to be researched. The various concepts of the specific question are made operational. Thus it becomes clear which data is to be collected, in what manner it is to be collected and from whom. In the next phase, possibly preceded by a pilot study, the data are collected and processed with analytical techniques established in advance. In the research report the findings are finally recorded and related to the theoretical starting points.

Possible conclusions are drawn. Mention may also be made of points for further discussion and recommendations for further research.

3

QUALITATIVE RESEARCH

3.1 INTRODUCTION

Western science, characterised by rationalism and empiricism distinguishes between a 'real world' which can be observed and a 'world of perceptions, beliefs and experiences'. Rational knowledge is believed to emerge out of reasoning based on the principles of logic while according to empiricism knowledge is produced empirically i.e. by observing phenomena through the human senses. Cause and effect relationships form the focus of this scientific form of enquiry. Universal laws are 'deducted' or drawn up to explain, predict and control phenomena. After going through a process of falsification and/or verification these laws or theories can be generalised to similar phenomena, transcending time and cultural boundaries. New theories emerge or others are refined through this process of falsification and verification (see Chapter 1).

The methodology of rational empiricism, also referred to as logical empiricism, depends on operational definitions, measurement and statistical analysis in order to produce knowledge. This approach to research is characteristic of the natural sciences.

3.2 POSITIVISM

With the emergence of Positivism, a school of thought founded by Auguste Comte, it was believed that the same research principles can be applied to the social sciences. Howe (1988) describes Positivists as taking the view that scientific knowledge is the paragon of rationality and that
'...scientific knowledge must be free of metaphysics, that is, that it must be based on pure observation that is free of interests, values, purposes and psychological schemata of individuals; and that anything that deserves the name 'knowledge' including social science, of course, must measure up to these standards.'
For example, in the study of human behaviour, Positivists would observe particular behaviours without taking into account the meanings that humans give to their actions.

3.3 INTERPRETIVISM

Human behaviour can only be understood when the context in which it takes place and the cognitive processes which give rise to it are studied. According to Hughes (1976) 'men and women are not particles acted upon by exogenous forces; they are 'purposeful, goal-seeking, feeling, meaning-attributing and meaning-responding creatures'.'

It was a matter of time before alternative approaches to the rational empiricism emerged. The failure of Positivism to address the main focus of enquiry by using the most appropriate methodology gave rise to criticisms. Walker (1985) discerns two distinct but related themes in the writings of the critics of Positivism:
(a) that Positivistic social science research in its concern with scientific procedures, hypothesis testing, measurement, statistical significance and the like has become sterile and introspective; and
(b) that fundamental differences between the natural and social worlds rule out the possibility of using techniques of natural science to study social phenomena.

These alternative research approaches have been loosely labelled Interpretivism, mainly because researchers focus their enquiry on the interpretation of the actions and in the context in which they occur. Howe (1988) describes interpretivists as taking the view that, at least as far as the social sciences are concerned, metaphysics (in the form of human intentions, beliefs and so forth) cannot be eliminated; observation cannot be pure in the sense of altogether excluding interests, values, purposes and psychological schemata.

3.4 IDEAL TYPES

Positivism and Interpretivism 'reflect fundamentally different epistemologies concerning the sort of knowledge about the social world which it is possible to achieve and different philosophies as to the nature of man' (Walker, 1985). Oiler and Munhall (1986) emphasise the need to 'recognize these differences and to accept their irreconcilable nature'. Increasingly researchers are using concepts and methods from both paradigms to study the same phenomena. This mixing of traditions is encouraged by some (Howe, 1988) and discouraged by others (Leininger, 1992). The debate about whether the two paradigms are compatible or not is likely to continue for a long time. In reality a large number of research studies do not fit neatly into either tradition. It is useful, therefore, to treat each paradigm as ideal types with which research studies can be contrasted.

The ideal-type Positivist research paradigm can be described as follows:
– Knowledge is produced deductively. What is already known is 'tested' by further research. This is either rejected or modified to produce theories. New theories are tested again and the process continues.
– The techniques of data collection are highly structured. For example, measurements can be made with the use of thermometers or attitude scales.
– Values are attributed to observation units. For example, numbers may be assigned to different forms of behaviour being studied and the scores become central to the understanding of behaviour.
– The data collected are devoid of the biases of researchers and respondents. These data are termed 'hard' or objective, as they are amenable to statistical analyses.
– Research is carried out in a laboratory or simulated laboratory condition.

The ideal-type Interpretivist research paradigm can be described as follows:
– Knowledge is produced inductively. Concepts and theories emerge from observation and interpretation of phenomena.

– The techniques of data collection are unstructured, for example in-depth interviews and unstructured participant observation. The researcher collects and analyses data as the research progresses.

– The data collected are interpreted by the researcher and the respondents and have a high degree of subjectivity.

– Data are termed 'soft' since they take the form of description of conversations or diary notes and are not necessarily amenable to statistical analysis.

– Research is carried out in the contexts or situations in which phenomena occur.

3.5 QUALITATIVE RESEARCH

Research carried out in the interpretivist paradigm is called qualitative research. The latter has often been defined mainly according to the methodology used. Thus, Strauss and Corbin (1990) describe qualitative research as 'any kind of research that produces findings not arrived at by means of quantification.' Bogdan and Biklen (1982) offer another description of qualitative research:

'we use qualitative research as an umbrella term to refer to several research strategies that share certain characteristics. The data collected has been termed 'soft', that is rich in description of people, places, conversations and not easily handled by statistical procedures. Research questions are not framed by operationalizing variables; rather, they are formulated to investigate in all their complexity, in context.'

Qualitative research can also be said to share more or less the same foci of study. In contrast to positivistic research where observed behaviour is the focus of study, qualitative researchers study behaviour from the viewpoint of the actor and in the context in which action takes place.

Although qualitative researchers may be described as sharing a humanistic philosophy, their beliefs, as reflected in their research, are shaped by the particular branch of the discipline from which they operate.

3.6 QUALITATIVE VERSUS QUANTITATIVE

Research carried out in the positivist paradigm is often termed quantitative. It is sometimes believed that the difference between quantitative and qualitative research is that the former deals with quantity and the latter with quality. Certainly positivist researchers tend to use large samples, structured measuring instruments, and analyse their data statistically. But many qualitative researchers use some form of quantification when analysing their data. Atkinson et al (1988) maintain that 'in a deeper sense, almost all qualitative research involves quantitative claims, albeit expressed in verbal rather than in numerical form.' The increasing use of computers allows for more elaborate and sophisticated analysis of qualitative data although numerical values may or may not be assigned to such data. One of the most commonly used packages is 'Ethnograph'.

Qualitative purists may frown upon the use of statistical or mathematical formulas in qualitative research. The difference between quantitative and qualitative research is not so much that one uses statistical methods and the other does not, but rather that in quantitative research numerical values are central to the understanding of phenomena, while in qualitative research they are either incidental or of no importance.

3.7 QUALITATIVE RESEARCH TERMINOLOGIES.

There are a number of terms which are frequently used in qualitative research literature. Some of these are used interchangeably. It would be impossible for scholars from the same country, let alone from different countries, to agree on the meanings of all the terms used. Different intellectual cultures and historical periods have coined their own terminologies. The reader, however, must seek to understand the specific meaning which the author attributes to particular terms.

Among the terms which cause most confusion are paradigms, tradition, approach and method. Paradigms and traditions are sometimes used to describe the same concept. For example Oiler and Munhall (1986) contrast Kuhn's(1970) definition of a paradigm 'as a discipline's specific method of solving a puzzle, of viewing human experience, and of structuring reality' and Laudan's(1977) description of a research tradition as a set of assumptions about the basic kinds of entities in the world, assumptions about how these entities interact, assumptions about the proper methods to use for constructing and testing theories about these entities. Oiler and Munhall found that both authors are conveying the same meaning. A paradigm tends to be defined as the overall philosophical framework of how scientific knowledge is produced. Any deviation from it means that the researcher is using another paradigm. Tradition seems to be a term used to describe research using more or less the same type of methodologies.

Approaches and methods are also used interchangeably. It is not unusual to find that some authors use the term 'phenomenological approach' while others use 'phenomenological method' to mean the same thing. Approaches and methods are sometimes used to describe the overall methodology. A number of approaches such as phenomenology and grounded theory specify the different steps or stages that researchers should adopt when using these particular theoretical orientations. Methods seem to signify adhesion to particular rules and guidelines while approaches embody an element of informality and flexibility within a set of rules. The term 'qualitative methods' is often used to describe the techniques of data collection such as in-depth interviews and participant observation.

A dogmatic use of research terminologies can lead to frustration. It suffices that the author is clear about the meaning, and is consistent in his or her use of research terminologies.

STUDY ACTIVITY 1

You have decided to study interactions between nurses and patients. What aspects of these interactions would you select for your investigation ? Consider the strengths and limitations of a qualitative approach for this study.

3.8 MAIN APPROACHES IN QUALITATIVE RESEARCH

There are four main approaches or methods in qualitative research and these are phenomenology, symbolic interactionism, ethnography and grounded theory.

3.8.1 Phenomenology

Phenomenology can be said to underpin all qualitative research because it focuses on individuals' interpretation of their own experiences. In fact it is not unusual to find that when some authors write about qualitative research they are in fact only writing about the phenomenological method.

Phenomenology is a branch of philosophy. To fully understand it one has to read the original work of Husserl (1965), its founding father. Amongst other philosophers who have made valuable contributions to phenomenology are Merleau-Ponty (1964) and Sartre (1963).

'Phenomenology may be regarded as a different way of looking at traditional philosophical problems such as the concept of the self, free will, one's body, perception, values, language and metaphysics.' (Emden, 1991). Researchers using the phenomenological approach are concerned about how individuals and groups perceive their worlds. We often find it hard to understand why people see things differently from us. How individuals and groups experience and interpret what happens to them and around them differ from setting to setting. One of the concerns of health professionals is the phenomenon of non-compliance of laymen with professional advice. The phenomenological method has the potential of discovering the reasons why this is so, by studying how people view professional advice and how this advice fits into their social and beliefs systems.

For the phenomenologist, the perceived world is the real world (Stewart and Mickunas, 1974). Actions and language reveal more than what they appear to convey. The task of phenomenologists is to uncover the various conscious and unconscious ways in which humans express themselves and how they 'live' their experiences.

Baker et al (1992) explain that consciousness is intentional and that the object of phenomenological enquiry is the description of the phenomena as experienced by the individual. According to them reduction consists of the researcher divesting himself of herself of preconceptions and of exploring the various ways respondents experience this phenomenon which then leads to the uncovering of the essential structure i.e. the essence of the phenomenon experienced.

Because phenomenologists are interested in the views of respondents, it is sometimes wrongly believed that some open- ended questions or a semi-structured interview would constitute the phenomenological method. For the latter to be used properly the whole methodology of a study should be conceived in the phenomenological tradition. The phenomenological method or approach consists of a set of steps or stages which guide researchers in the study of phenomena. Spiegelberg (1976) writes about seven steps of the phenomenological method which include 'investigating particular phenomena', 'investigating general essences' and 'apprehending

41

essential relationships and essences'. Van Kaam (1959) in his study of 'really being understood' uses five steps as does Paterson and Zderad (1976) although the latter's steps are not the same as Van Kaam's.

Phenomenological researchers also differ on which aspects of the research process to concentrate. Some, like Spiegelberg (1976) lay emphasis on the 'emancipation from preconceptions', others like Giorgi (1971) concentrate on data analysis.

However, there are perhaps as many different phenomenological methodologies as there are phenomenological researchers. The strength of qualitative research is that researchers can bend the approach to study phenomena rather than the other way round. It is also important to stress that there are different interpretations of phenomenology.

The techniques of data collection include participant observation in the natural environment, indepth or unstructured interview and diary recording. These techniques are described in Section 3.11.

The importance of phenomenology to nursing and other health professionals is explained by Wilkes (1991):
'Practice is a 'lived-experience' and as such involves not only the nurse but other health professionals and at the centre the client (the nursed). It involves human beings experiencing and interacting'.
Using a phenomenological approach can help nurses to understand, for example what 'health' or 'caring' means to the client. This approach may lead to the development of concepts and themes which in turn can be applied to practice.

Examples of phenomenological research
An exploratory design using phenomenological analysis was applied to understand the female registered nurses' experiences of nursing patients throughout the lifespan and to uncover behaviours commonly believed nurturant (Geissler, 1990).

Anderson's (1991) inquiry into existential experience of illness in a group of immigrant women begins from a phenomenological perspective and proceeds to examine the context in which experiences are embedded.

3.8.2 Symbolic Interactionism.
As explained above, phenomenology underpins most other forms of qualitative research in that it studies participants' worldview. There are also other theories which seek to explain human behaviour. One which is frequently used is symbolic interactionism. It focuses on the meanings of events to people and the symbols they use to convey that meaning (Baker et al, 1992). According to Blumer (1969) there are three premises on which symbolic interactionism rests. These are:

1. A human being acts towards things on the basis of the meanings that the things have for him.

2. Meaning of such things is derived from or arises out of social interaction that one has with one's fellows.

3. These meanings are handled in and modified through an interpretative process by the person in dealing with the things he encounters.

People use symbols to structure their world. Apart from the rituals and ceremonies which contain obvious symbols, there are many symbols inherent in everyday interactions. A symbol is simply the meaning that an event or action has apart from their obvious functional use. For example lighting a cigarette is not only a response to a physical or psychological craving but may also signify the completion of a task. A cigarette at the end of a meal marks the completion of the ritual of eating. The process of constantly interpreting, and reacting to these symbols is called symbolic interactionism. It is a belief that there is a physical and a social as well as a psychological constructed environment. People react not only to physical stimuli but also as a result of how they perceive the social environment.

Central to the understanding of symbolic interactionism is the concept of self. As Bogdan and Biklen (1982) explain

> 'The self is the definition people create (through interacting with others) of who they are. In constructing or defining self, people attempt to see themselves as others see them by interpreting gestures and actions directed toward them and by placing themselves in the role of the other person. In short we come to see ourselves in part as others see us.'

Symbolic interactionism tries to explain the process of how meanings are arrived at or conceived by individuals in their everyday interactions as compared to phenomenology which seeks only to describe the essence of human experience. The notion is best explicated by George Herbert Mead (1934), who is recognised as the founding father of American social psychology and the originator of that branch of sociology known as symbolic interactionism. Mead's now famous idea of 'taking the role of the other' is central to the symbolic interactionist approach. He claimed that we take our role from the 'generalized other' by behaving in accordance with how we perceive others as expecting us to behave. Thus the self is a product of interaction within the social situation.

It must be recognised that to some extent symbolic interactionists and phenomenologists share an interest in the influence of the social situation. The phenomenological sociologist Alfred Schutz (1972) has also drawn attention to the influence of others on how we think and feel, when he states that :

> 'Every act of mine through which I endow the world with meaning refers back to some meaning-endowing act ... of yours with respect to the same world. Meaning is thus constituted as an intersubjective phenomenon.'

This notion is very similar to Mead's (op. cit.) idea of 'taking the role of the other'. The essential difference is that phenomenologists are primarily interested in the deep subjective meanings we attribute to, and the experiences we feel towards, particular objects. While there are many influences on the meanings we attribute to objects, in the end it is the individual who confers his own meaning upon them by a process of 'intentionality'. We intend to, or decide to, see something as having a particular meaning and it thus in the end is 'subjective', or the subject of our attention, rather than an objective reality. This is fundamentally different to the symbolic interactionist perspective, which sees the individual almost as a tabula rasa, whose understandings and attributed meanings, and the behaviour which results, arise to a large extent from his/her interactions with others. They are thus social constructions of reality rather than individual constructions dependent upon intentionality (see, for example, Berger and Luckmann, 1967).

STUDY ACTIVITY 2

Observe how a nurse in a ward in your hospital behaves. Make a brief summary of her role behaviours. Then identify the other people with whom the nurse interacts. Try to identify the expectations these people have of the nurse and explain the extent to which the nurse you have selected conforms or does not conform to these expectations. Conclude with a view on how this nurse has been influenced by Mead's process of 'taking the role of the other'.

(You have done a little piece of qualitative research! Write it up in about 500 words and file it with your course notes.)

The sociological symbolic interactionist perspective conceives of reality as dynamic rather than static and it focuses on processes that exist within the individual or groups of individuals rather than on social structure (Baker et al 1992). Thus in a doctor-patient relationship the behaviour of the patient is not only explained in terms of the power relationship between the two but also according to how the patient views the doctor (taking into account various variables, such as gender, age, position in society) apart from the obvious role of healer. This patient also reacts according to how she thinks the doctor views her and how he or she (i.e. the doctor) is seen to expect the patient to behave. The phenomenologist would be more concerned with the patient's experience, i.e. the outcome rather than the process of this relationship. Symbolic interaction focuses on interactions and as such is appropriate in understanding nursing phenomena where interactions are the main features. Phenomenology with its emphasis on experience is more appropriate for the study of phenomena where the individual experience is the focal point, bearing in mind that in all human experience, the concept of interaction is present.

The techniques of data collection for those using this approach include participant observation, in-depth interview and analysis of written materials such as diaries and autobiographies. Symbolic interactionists have different views of the role of this method in relation to the generation of theories. Some would perhaps see theories as emerging from the data collected rather than use data to verify or test theories (Bogdan and Taylor 1975). Others like Blumer (1969) sees the symbolic interactionist method as producing theories which can thereafter be empirically verified.

Examples of research underpinned by symbolic interactionism
Simmons (1990) used symbolic interactionism to study 'what psychiatric illness means to carers in the community'. With the use of guided interview format she

explored the meanings of some of the issues for those who find themselves in the position of caring for someone with a mental health problem in the community. Cowley (1991) in a study examining the role of health visitors in health promotion adopted a symbolic interactionist approach to analyse the interactions between health visitors and their clients. Porter (1991), with the use of participant observations, researched how nurse-doctor power relations are manifested in a hospital setting. He based the design of this project on symbolic interactionism because the latter 'asserts that reality, rather than being a fixed entity, is continually being recreated by the meaningful actions and interactions of social actions'.

The researcher – researched relationship itself would benefit from a symbolic interactionist analysis of the interactions between the two. An understanding of how the participant views the researcher and how the former presents himself or herself would shed more light on the validity and reliability of the data.

3.8.3 Ethnography

Ethnography is more of a method or approach than an underlying philosophy. Ethnographers believe that phenomena can only be understood if studied in the context in which they happen. Therefore researchers can use concepts from phenomenology, symbolic interactionism and grounded theory (see 3.8.4 below) in order to study people in the social and cultural environment in which they live and work. However, while phenomenological and symbolic interactionist approaches tend to be derived from existential philosophy and the humanistic sociology tradition, ethnography is essentially from an entirely different tradition, that of social anthropology which is concerned with the culture and customs of groups of people. Jacob (1987) explains that the goal of ethnographers is to 'describe a unique way of life, documenting the meanings attached to events and showing how the parts fit together into an integrated whole.'

Ethnographers place particular emphasis on studying groups and communities as a unified whole. According to them, individuals, groups, families, religion, ceremonies, social organisations, economic systems interrelate to produce a cultural environment. No part can, therefore, be studied and understood on its own.

Ethnography is a branch of anthropology, and early European and American researchers studied mainly tribes and villagers in far away places. Doing 'fieldwork' used to mean going abroad to live in these communities in order to collect and analyse data. In modern times, ethnographers have looked closer to home for topics of enquiry. Thus ethnographic research has taken place in a wide variety of physical and social environments that include the 'corporate boardroom, the classroom, the hospital operating room, the physician's waiting room, the intensive care unit in a modern hospital, the retirement nursing home' (Hughes, 1992).

One of the central features and strengths of the ethnographic approach is that the researcher must as far as possible immerse himself or herself in the culture under study. Hence, the term 'going native' was coined to describe a researcher who tries to integrate into the community and take part in the activities in which his or her subjects engage . In this way the researcher is able to experience the world of his or her subjects. The term often used to describe this phenomenon is 'emic' i.e. where the researcher endeavours to experience phenomena as his or her subjects experience these phenomena, as opposed to 'etic' i.e. where the researcher imposes meaning on the experience of his or her subjects. However, during ethnographic fieldwork the researcher has the opportunity to observe these phenomena from his or her own perspective as well, since no one can go totally 'native'. In this way the ethnographer sees the world from both sides.

There are many offshoots of ethnography. Field and Morse (1985) include ethnology and ethnoscience in their lists. Jacob (1987) writes about ethnology of communication. While it is not the purpose of this chapter to describe these variations on, or extensions of, the ethnographic theme, it is important when reading research reports or articles to understand the concepts and methods which are used rather than getting into dogmatic discussions on labelling.

The techniques of collecting and analysing data may vary according to different forms of ethnography. However, mainstream ethnography uses participant observation as well as unstructured interviews to gather data. Since the whole culture is under study the ethnographer is interested in various aspects of culture such as art, music, language, literature etc.. All these are valuable sources of information.

Ethnography as a research approach is becoming more popular in nursing and health. Hughes (1992) wonders whether this is 'simply a passing fancy, a fad comparable to fashion styles or transitory language habits'. However, nursing provides many cultural environments which are eminently amenable to ethnographic research.

Examples of ethnographic research
Millman (1975) studied the 'backrooms' of American medicine by observing ' what was said and done in operating rooms, and at Mortality Review Conferences in the Emergency room and at various kinds of hospital staff meetings'. In her two-year long study using non-participant unstructured observations, she was 'able to get a feeling for the texture and quality of staff life in a hospital'.
Aamodt (1984) using one kind of ethnographic methodology focused on a 'child's view of chemically induced alopecia'.

Sometimes published texts can reveal ethnographic traits. Ruffing-Rahal (1991) analysed the writings of Mary Brekinridge and found that the latter gave very full accounts of people in their physical, social and cultural contexts of everyday life: 'As ethnographic texts, Brekinridge's writings are the strategic recollections of a culturally informed nurse in organizing district systems of health care'.

3.8.4 Grounded theory
Grounded theory in its simplest form means theory which emerges out of data grounded in the observation and interpretation of phenomena. Strauss and Corbin (1990) describe grounded theory 'as a qualitative research method that uses a

systematic set of procedures to develop an inductively derived grounded theory about a phenomenon'.

Developed by Glaser and Strauss (1967) its systematic techniques and procedures of analysis enable the researcher to develop a substantive theory that meets the criteria for doing 'good' science: significance, theory - observation compatibility, general-isability, reproducibility, precision rigour, and verification. Readers interested in the grounded theory method should consult the original work of Glaser and Strauss (1967) for their original exposé of these concepts. Although according to Baker (1992) grounded theory is rooted in the symbolic interactionist school of sociology, Strauss and Corbin (1990) maintain that this method 'can be used by persons of any discipline or theoretical orientation desirous of developing a grounded theory'. A perusal of research literature reveals that many researchers interpret grounded theory simply as an inductive method to produce knowledge and use various theoretical orientations to study phenomena.

Grounded theory emerged as an alternative approach to the deductive method of producing knowledge. Grounded theory is useful in that it allows researchers to 'start afresh' and not to be influenced by the present knowledge about certain phenomena. Many scientific discoveries have been made by the accidental spilling of chemical solutions on the laboratory table,which made scientists realise that their approaches are sometimes wrong. Constrained by its rigid laws, the dominant paradigm (Posi-tivism) can produce scientists who think alike. What is required are people who can devise new ways of thinking about phenomena. The inductive method, on the other hand, as advocated by grounded theorists, starts from almost a clean slate. Its drawbacks are that it risks reinventing the wheel and also frustrate its followers who feel a sense of failure when theories do not emerge easily from the ground. Strauss and Corbin (1990) emphasise that it is only by practising the procedures of grounded theory through continued research that one gains sufficient understanding of how they work.

The techniques of data collection are the same as those in most other forms of qualitative research. The analysis of data is rigorous in that the researcher has to reflect on categories and test emerging concepts and theories many times before firm theoretical propositions can be made.

The potential value of grounded theory to the development of nursing science is great. As a new discipline, nursing has only begun to develop concepts and theories which can, in turn, influence practice. Most nursing research carried out has been in the positivistic paradigm. This may be because of the dominance of the medical model (itself an adherent to Positivism) and/or because of the scientific aura which quantitative research bestows on its followers.

Qualitative research, using a grounded theory approach, is however becoming more popular in the United Kingdom as evidenced by articles in research journals and by papers presented at research conferences. Leininger (1992) remarks that in the U.S.,'qualitative paradigmatic research has come of age and is being fully recognised as a legitimate, essential and important means to advance humanistic and scientific knowledge'.

Examples of research using the grounded theory method
Keller (1991) used a grounded theory approach to explore the post-operative experiences of patients following coronary bypass surgery. Data collection took place over nine months and consisted of ten unstructured, interactive interviews resulting in over 400 pages of transcriptions. The researcher also asked the respondents to describe their experience of coronary artery bypass from the onset of symptoms and entry to the healthcare system and continued through the post-operative recovery period (Keller 1991).

Dowd (1991) studied older women's experience of urinary incontinence. As she explained it 'discovering grounded theory was chosen as the method of enquiry because it allows for the expansion of knowledge based on the study of human experience as it is lived'. It is clear that phenomenology underpins her study although she does not mention it.

3.9 DIVERSITY IN USE OF QUALITATIVE APPROACHES

As more and more research is carried out in the qualitative paradigm it is becoming clear that many researchers are eclectic in their use of approaches. What is clearer, however, is that some researchers are adopting a reductionist approach to the use of phenomenology and grounded theory. It is not uncommon to find that in cases where respondents are simply asked their views that the research approach has been termed 'phenomenological'. Similarly grounded theory is taken to mean simply using an inductive approach to research.

Some researchers do not reveal the assumptions underpinning their methodologies while others report adopting an approach which seems to be different from what is described in the report. A certain degree of caution must be exerted when reading research reports which do not make clear which approaches are used and how.

3.10 THE PROCESS OF QUALITATIVE RESEARCH

The various approaches described above have their own method or framework which guide the research process. It is difficult to generalise about the research process in qualitative research because by definition this type of research is flexible. Researchers can use their imagination and creativity in devising the most appropriate methodologies in the study of phenomena. However, this flexibility should not be at the expense of application and rigour.

Positivistic research has distinct stages of the research process, although the actual stages are not as neatly distinguishable as the research reports suggest. Qualitative research stages are not necessarily linear; often researchers go back to previous stages before proceeding further. Thus it is not unusual for researchers after an initial analysis of data to go back to respondents in order to clarify interpretations. Some researchers may also decide to go back to the literature once data have been collected.

Others choose not to be influenced and consult the literature only at the end (see Chapter 5).

Most qualitative research involves a degree of reflection and introspection by the researcher, followed by a stage in which the researcher is open to all perspectives, during which most of the data are collected and terminating with the researcher using his or her own skills, knowledge and experience to analyse the data. In practice these stages are sometimes not followed nor easily recognisable in the research reports.

The researcher in qualitative research is the tool of data collection and analysis, although other techniques are used to supplement these functions. The researcher must be able to be critical and analytical of the data as these are being collected. Further analysis takes place later on. One important aspect of the researcher which is often neglected in the discussion of research is the personality of the researcher. There is little doubt that access to information as well as trust-building between researcher and researched often depend on the 'person' of the researcher. This either facilitates or hinders the research process and may even affect the validity and reliability of the findings.

3.11 TECHNIQUES OF DATA COLLECTION

According to Lincoln (1992) there are two kinds of qualitative data collection techniques: human-to-human and artifactual. The first refers to such techniques as interviewing and observation and the second refers to the analysis and examination of artifacts such as written materials (e.g. biographies, letters, diaries etc.) or artistic expressions such as paintings, music, sculptures etc.

Qualitative techniques are mainly unstructured and contextual. Positivistic research depends on the precision of the instruments and therefore uses highly structured ones. However, in social research, despite the use of carefully constructed instruments, the validity of the data is sometimes questionable. The survey, a much used positivistic tool, has serious limitations in studying behaviour. Mechanic (1989) explains that while the social survey makes efforts to measure important contextual variables it 'typically separates most behaviour measured from the particular historical, social and cultural contexts in which it is embedded'. Three main techniques of qualitative data collection will be described here. These are unstructured observations, indepth interviews and artifactual analyses.

3.11.1 Unstructured observations

Unstructured observations are so-called because, while the area of enquiry is known, the particular research question/s which the researcher will pursue may only become clear after the researcher enters the field. As Mechanic (1989) explains

> 'what the researcher selects as important from an almost infinite number of possible observations, and how each observation ...(is weighted in relation to)... others in a larger organising frame of reference, determine to a major extent the construction that emerges.'

49

Studying the interpretation of participants requires an open-ended approach to observations. Although most researchers have an idea of what to observe, they find that they are soon attracted to certain phenomena more than others. Millman (1975) using unstructured observations describes how she became interested in certain issues:

> 'At first my research interests were quite general. I soon found, however, that my attentions were drawn toward two intriguing issues. One was the variety of ways that doctors define, perceive and respond to medical mistakes ... the second major issue I came to focus on is the competing interests and conflicts among various groups of doctors within the hospital'.

3.11.2 Participant and non-participant observation

These two types of observation are at the opposite end of a continuum according to Gold (1958). *Non-participant observation* is when the researcher does not take part in the activities of his subjects. By observing but not participating he hopes to obtain an accurate and uncontaminated record of what is happening. However the mere presence of the observer may affect what is being observed, except if observation takes place via a one-way mirror or screen and the participants are totally unaware of it, or if the researcher is using covert approaches. This mere presence effect has also been described as reactivity (Webb et al, 1966) and observer interference (Weick, 1968). It has been suggested that the mere presence or reactivity effect is transitory and that after a brief period subjects forget or choose to overlook the fact that they are being observed and behave normally (Posner, 1980). However, in a review of research dealing with reactivity, Johnson and Bolstad (1973) found that in some cases there was a major reactivity effect while in others this was not the case. They suggest that the main factors were:
  – the consciousness of the observer;
  – personal characteristics of the subjects;
  – personal characteristics of the observer;
  – reason given to subjects for observing.

Sometimes, if the researcher is not a practitioner but wants to study aspects of the practitioners' life, the *non-participant observation* method can be very useful. Millman (1975) carried out non-participant observations in a hospital and found that she was able to 'observe how the various groups of doctors viewed and gave meaning to the situations which arose, and how they chose to pay attention to some things and not to others.'

In order to have a fuller understanding of the experience of respondents, which is the purpose of qualitative research, the researcher must immerse himself or herself in the activities of those being studied. In other words, the researcher does not stand apart (as in non-participant observation) but becomes a member of the group. This is *participant observation*. In some instances the researcher negotiates his/her participant observer status openly. However, in other cases this is done covertly. The researcher enters the scene e.g. as just another student (in a college) or worker (in the workplace) and no one, or perhaps only the senior management, know that he or she is a researcher. This greatly reduces the mere presence influence. However, there are also important ethical considerations here and in some situations e.g. in prisons or in subcultural settings - with racist groups or drug abusers - the approach may be very dangerous.

Participant observation is particularly important in ethnographic and phenomenological studies. It gives the researcher the opportunity not only to observe what happens but also to experience to some extent certain aspects of the lives of other people. This requires a high degree of empathy in the researcher.

Participant and non-participant observers normally take notes in diary and memo format and reflect on these as they progress with the research. When reading research reports it is important to understand the context in which the observations were made, how the data were recorded and the subjective selection and interpretation of phenomena under study.

3.11.3 Interviews in qualitative research

Most of the interviews carried out in qualitative research can be described as 'unstructured' or 'indepth' or 'depth'. Interviewing can be the main data collection technique or it can be used to accompany observations. As Millman (1975) explains:

> 'Because I was present for such a long time, I was able not only to observe their behaviour (physicians) but I could also ask physicians about their thoughts and feelings in the course of ongoing events.'

Understanding the experience of respondents requires a degree of freedom to verbalise their thoughts without the researcher imposing his or her views and wishes on them. Unstructured interviews therefore allow the respondents the flexibility on what is said. Qualitative researchers vary in the amount of direction they want to give to the interview process, and therefore this dictates the extent of control which interviewers have on the interview process. Interviewers in qualitative research require skills not only to encourage the respondent to talk but also skills to assimilate what is being said. As Hedges (1985) points out

'He or she will have to make decisions throughout the interview as to whether a given line of enquiry is proving useful and worth pursuing, or fruitless and to be headed off - and this has to be done in the light of his understanding of the problem and hence of the possible relevance or irrelevance of particular kinds of information.'

To understand the interpretations of respondents' experiences it is sometimes necessary to carry out more than one interview with the same respondent. For example Anderson (1991) in a study of the experience of chronic illness among immigrant women carried out an average of three in-depth ethnographic interviews lasting from one to one and a half hours each with the women in the sample at approximately six-monthly intervals.

In quantitative research each interview must have the same content and must be carried out in the same way each time it is repeated. This is not necessarily the case in qualitative interviews. For example, the last interviewee may be asked different questions from the first one. Dowd (1991) explains how her interviews were modified during the process of her research into older women's experience of urinary incontinence:

> 'Data collection processes were modified as new information was gathered and new avenues for exploration were uncovered. For example, in the first interviews the women were asked to describe an accident they had had. However, the third respondent denied having any accidents, but instead described her experience with urinary incontinence and how she managed to prevent any accidents from occurring. The interviewer then modified the question by asking subsequent respondents to describe their experience with urinary incontinence'.

With qualitative interviews the researcher is not mainly concerned with how many people subscribes to a particular perspective or viewpoint, but in the different perspectives which respondents hold. Data in unstructured interviews can be recorded on audio tape or in notes form. The free flow of information often depends on how unobtrusive the recording is.

STUDY ACTIVITY 3
A researcher has used a questionnaire to investigate leadership styles on a number of surgical wards. What other methods would you use and why ?

3.11.4 Artifactual analysis
To have a holistic view of the experience of the respondents all forms of expression must be examined. The most obvious and useful source of information apart from direct observation and interviews are written materials whether in the form of books, leaflets, diaries, memos, or letters.

However, artifacts do not necessarily have to be written materials. They may be photographs, clothing, tools – almost any man-made objects. The subjects themselves do not have to be present. Indeed, in some instances they may have left the scene. They may even be dead, and all that remains is their letters or diaries. Where subjects are still in the setting, there is also often the possibility that they are unaware (at least until afterwards) that such data is being collected, thus reducing mere presence or reactivity effects. Good examples of this can be found in the literature describing unobtrusive measures (see for example, Webb et al. 1966). Such research has involved, for example, analysing the contents of waste baskets in office buildings or doing counts of empty alcohol bottles in neighbourhood garbage containers to establish alcohol consumption levels. Unobtrusive measures are of course covert methods and raise the same ethical questions identified in the section on observations above. For example, doing counts of cigarettes ends, crisp bags, chocolate wrappers, discarded magazines etc. in rest rooms may give interesting insights into nurses rest period activities. However, the subjects may subsequently take great offence at how their privacy was infringed in this way. Such ethical questions are of major concern to all who embark upon the research process and of equal concern to those who grant access to researchers or who agree to become subjects in a research project.

STUDY ACTIVITY 4

If you tell subjects exactly what you are researching it may significantly modify their behaviour and negate your research. If you do not tell the subjects, or if you observe them covertly without their permission, reactivity effects are unlikely, but there is a major ethical problem. Go to the college library and do literature searches and read-ups on the following topics:
– the meaning of 'ethics';
– the notion of 'informed consent';
– the 'unobtrusive measures' approach.

Spend two or three hours on this, over a few days if necessary. Then write an essay of one thousand words, quoting relevant references, on the topic: 'The justification for using unobtrusive measures'. Keep the essay for further reflection and study and if possible ask your personal tutor/supervisor to read it and discuss it with you.

Artistic expressions in the form of songs, dance, sculpture, music, literature etc. also provide a unique insight into peoples lives. The researcher, however, needs to be skillful in order to unravel the cognitive processes in the formulation of such expressions.

3.12 WORKING IN THE FIELD

Qualitative researchers need a set of attitudes to accompany their knowledge, skills and experience. Overwhelming the respondent with a dazzling display of knowledge may be counter-productive, as is adopting the position of an inquisitive investigator. The position of a confident learner is perhaps one that best befits the researcher. After all, one carries out such research in order to learn about people. Bogdan and Biklen (1982) succinctly capture the essence of the researchers role:

'Becoming a researcher means internalising the research goal while collecting data in the field. As you conduct research you participate with the subjects in various ways. You joke with them and behave sociably in many ways. You may even help them perform their duties. You do these things, but always for the reason of promoting your research goals.'

When the researcher enters the field, he or she is faced with having to decide how to behave. Often researchers are conscious, indeed oversensitive, to the mere presence effect referred to earlier. They are (usually) alone and they are outsiders. In the very act of being self-conscious and being concerned about mere presence or observer interference they may draw attention to themselves unduly and introduce those effects in what almost amounts to a self-fulfilling prophecy. This tendency to over-react to the research environment has been documented by Sanders (1980):

'... observation is not an approach with which all researchers are equally comfortable .... A natural and common experience is the fear which arises from finding oneself to be a stranger in the home territory of a group of actors bound by common understanding, strategies and problems .... This fear has its

53

foundation in the salient proscriptions we have learned concerning the illegitimacy of asking people probing questions .... In violating these rules, we risk personal rejection (and) not only does the field research appear to violate some deeply held rules of interaction, it also thrusts the researcher into an intensely self-conscious situation .... the result of critical focusing of attention on self.'

There is the danger of the researcher being preoccupied with his/her own at-risk situation, rather than being immersed in the field, the subjects and the data being collected. This danger extends beyond the risk of actually creating mere presence or observer interference effects. The researcher may become so apprehensive that his/her judgement becomes clouded and the data recorded is inaccurate or un-sound. Doing qualitative research is thus more than having the right inquisitive attitude. It is also about being controlled, and relaxed, and at ease in the field. And it is about the high levels of social skill involved in watching or asking questions which could be taken as offensive in an inoffensive manner.

3.13 ANALYSIS OF QUALITATIVE DATA

The main qualitative approaches such as the phenomenological method and the grounded theory method have guidelines for the analysis of data. For most types of qualitative research the data are already assimilated by the researchers during fieldwork. The notes taken or the audio tapes are transcribed and ready for analysis. While some researchers treat part of their data quantitatively, this is frowned upon by the qualitative purists. The use of computers in the analysis of qualitative data does not mean that the data are necessarily subjected to statistical analysis. Software packages are available for thematic qualitative analysis as well.

Jones (1985) explains that the analysis of qualitative data 'is a process of making sense, of finding and making a structure in the data and giving this meaning and signifi-cance for ourselves, and for any relevant audiences. As with data collection method-ologies, the way we do this and the kind of structures we look for in the data depend on the purpose of enquiry and what we see as the underlying purpose of qualitative research.' This means that different approaches have different forms of analysis. The most common treatment given to qualitative data is to structure them in themes or categories. For example, in Aamodt's (1986) study of alopecia, four culturally relevant themes emerged. These were 'There's nothing to be done','Loss of hair and loss of friends,' 'Getting used to it,' and 'Treat me as normal'.

In qualitative research each perspective or category is treated as important and may be explored further, while in positivistic research data are made to fit pre-existing categories and the most frequent categories emerge as important. The researcher looks for inconsistencies in the data as well and may return to the respondents for further validation of the data. There are other analytical methods such as cognitive mapping which is a method of modelling subjects' beliefs in diagrammatic form (Jones, 1985). Ingenuity and intuition in devising new, or adapting existing, suitable methods are the hallmarks of a good qualitative researcher. Whatever the methods used, the onus is on the researcher to provide detailed information to enable the reader to understand how the findings are arrived at.

3.14 VALIDITY AND RELIABILITY

Qualitative research is reckoned to be low on reliability and high on validity, while it is sometimes suggested that quantitative research is low on validity and high on reliability. It stands to reason that reliability without validity is of no great value. As Deutscher (1966) points out:

'we concentrate on consistency without much concern with what it is we are being consistent about or whether we are consistently right or wrong. As a consequence we have been learning a great deal about how to pursue an incorrect cause with a maximum of precision.'

The qualitative researcher can select subjectively what is to be observed or the questions to be asked. The loose framework of the research allows the researcher to follow his or her own intuition in deciding what to focus on. The analysis of qualitative data can also be highly subjective. Different researchers may not only use different analytical methods but are likely to come to different conclusions as well. Qualitative researchers may make their findings more objective by making their data available for others to analyse. However, although standardised questions or observations are thought to be more reliable methods of collecting data, according to Mechanic (1989) 'any experienced researcher knows that how one frames a question and selects response categories substantially affects the answers received.'

Siedman (1977) explains that the qualitative researcher considers various influences explicitly in his analysis in a way that the positivist rarely does. The author points out that '...few have questioned the inherent subjectivity of quantification which requires 'selection' of parameters and baseline data, the interpretation of findings, and the selection of facts and evidence. There is much to be gained by destroying the myth of objectivity since subjectivity is always intricately involved but disallowed'.

The question of the validity and reliability of qualitative research must be considered at a philosophical level as well. According to Leininger (1992), the goals of qualitative research are not to measure something but rather to understand fully the meaning of the phenomena under study. She further pointed out that the criteria for assessing reliability and validity are devised from the logical positivists' philosophical framework and are markedly different from qualitative criteria. The goal of positivistic research is to produce causal laws generalisable across cultures and throughout time. Qualitative research is about studying the particular at a specific time in history.

According to Lincoln and Guba (1985), ' the issue in any qualitative research is not whether another investigator would discover the same concepts to describe or interpret the data but whether the findings of an inquiry are worth paying attention to.' Positivistic researchers in the social sciences do not seem to have been very successful in generalising their findings to other similar phenomena. In fact many researchers in the quantitative tradition seem to caution against generalising from their results.

It should not be assumed from the above comments that qualitative researchers do not concern themselves with verifying their data. While they do not concern themselves with reliability (i.e. the extent to which findings can be repeated in different, but similar situations) they do, as indicated above, concern themselves with validity (i.e. ensuring that the data being analysed truly represents what it claims to represent). However, they do not conceive of validity in terms of statistical conclusion, as is the case with quantitative researchers. Instead they use more evaluative techniques, three of the most common being as follows:

Content validity. This is a value judgment which claims to confirm that the data presents what it truly claims to present. This includes *face validity* where an intuitive judgment is made that the data collected accurately reflects the true real-life situation. This depends of course on who is making the intuitive judgment. At its most dependable level, content validity is called *Expert validity.* There the researcher asks experts in the particular field to give judgments about the veracity of the data and analysis. Thus, experienced qualitative researchers may be asked if the method used is valid for collecting the data required and these researchers plus subjects or experts in the field of study can be asked to evaluate the content as a reflection of the real situation.

Presentation of rival explanations. Here the researcher seeks out all rival explanations for the data, weighs these against each other, and justifies that explanation which presents the 'best fit'. While using content validity or expert validity approaches, even where the researcher establishes a 'panel of experts', help to an extent, the nature of situation-specific qualitative data is such that only the researcher himself is immersed in the data. There is thus a need for the researcher himself to reflect upon all possible explanations, to step back from the data and look at 'the wood rather than the trees' and to focus on the most convincing explanation.

Consideration of negative cases. This includes attending not only to the cases which support the 'best fit' explanation, but also investigating the cases which do not support this stance. That is, the cases or subjects who drop out of the study, or those who present data which is in conflict with the proposed explanation.

Such techniques reflect a genuine concern for ensuring validity of analysis. However, it should be recognised, as suggested by Glaser and Strauss (1967) that there may be bias in the ways in which researchers seek out rival explanations or negative cases. Firstly, the researcher may reflect bias in terms of how arduously the rival explanations or negative cases are followed up and he or she may reflect a lack of open-mindedness in terms of willingness to review previous premises. Secondly the researcher may follow up rival explanations or negative cases using the same method e.g. in-depth interviewing. This may result in carrying methodological biases through to these checks for verification or validity. To avoid this threat to validity some researchers suggest a mixed method or triangulation approach throughout the research. That is, they use two or more qualitative methods to investigate the topic, on the assumption that biases in particular methods will be cancelled out. The issue of triangulation, including the assumption that biases can be cancelled out and the wider issue of mixing qualitative and quantitative methods, are discussed elsewhere in this text.

3.15 SUMMARY

In this chapter alternative approaches to the positivistic paradigm have been presented. They focus on the meanings that individual give to particular phenomena. The main approaches which were described were : phenomenology, symbolic interactionism, ethnography and grounded theory. The similarities, differences and methods have been highlighted. A summary of some of the main qualitative techniques of data collection and data analysis was offered. Finally, validity and reliability of qualitative research was briefly discussed.

4

THE RESEARCH PROBLEM

4.1 INTRODUCTION

An inquiry begins with a problem as its point of departure. As we have seen, various internal and external factors can stimulate research. In this chapter a number of typical problems and their origins will be discussed.

A clear definition of the problem seems the most obvious and self-evident activity in the research process, but it can be a source of difficulty in itself. This difficulty is closely connected with the nature of the scientific issue and the conditions set. These conditions will be discussed in this chapter.

4.2 PROBLEM IDENTIFICATION

4.2.1 Professional practice

An important source of research problems is experience. Everyday life in professional nursing practice contains many interesting problems. It can also be argued that professional practice ought, of necessity, to be subject to research, if nurses and others wish to be able to account for their actions as professionals. From this viewpoint it will be clear that those working in professional practice should be familiar with the various processes of research and should be able to identify problems from professional practice which might be suitable for scientific research.

There are various ways of arriving at scientific problems within professional practice:
  – via the nursing process. The nursing process continually requires explicit justification of the choices which the nurse makes with regard to patient care. Wherever these decisions take place on the basis of insufficient empirically verified knowledge, it can be stated that there is potential for scientific research;
  – there may be indications in the working environment pointing to research issues. For example, attention should be paid to the recurring every day comments, questions and frustrations that play a part within a team;
  – an alternative starting point might be found in the tension between the actual situation and that which is desirable. Specialised literature can provide further background about the problems that arise within professional practice.

STUDY ACTIVITY 1
From your own working experience, identify three subjects or issues on each of the three levels mentioned above, which might lead to scientific problems capable of research.

4.2.2 Theory

As will have become evident from Chapter 1, theorising is an important source of research problems. An important objective, especially in fundamental research, will be the verification of theory. The theory can be refined as a result of this type of research and thus gain in strength or be weakened or even rejected.

Example

In considering the phenomenon of nursing, scientific theories and models play an important part. In recent years theories about self care have become more and more popular. In practice it is of major importance that nurses are able to assess the degree of self-care properly, so that they can adjust nursing care to the needs of the patients. According to Orem's (1980) theory the sphere of nursing work lies where the self-care ability of people falls short of carrying out the necessary self-care behaviour.

The actions carried out by nurses to wholly or partially compensate for self care deficiencies, to give information and instructions and to guide and support patients in this, are called nursing actions. Orem distinguishes four kinds of functions, which together constitute the nursing process: diagnosing, planning actions, performing actions and evaluation. To be able to accomplish these functions, the nurse needs nursing skills.

Nursing proficiency is defined by Orem as follows.

It is the whole of knowledge and learning which we can find in the nurse(s) and a complex capacity to act, which is activated by nurses when they ascertain the need for nursing and determine the form of nursing intervention necessary among people with self care deficiencies.

An important assumption in Orem's theory about nursing actions is therefore the supposition that nurses are able to assess the self care capability of patients. The testing of this assumption for application of the theory in practice as well as in nursing and paramedical research is an important objective of research. After all, if nurses want to adapt their care to the needs of patients, they should be capable of assessing the self care ability of patients properly.

4.2.3 Research assignments

Provisional issues for research are also formulated on behalf of or by clients, such as a Health Authority or a patient interest group .

The provisional research question is comparable to the questions which nurses formulate from professional practice. Usually applied research is involved, intended to solve problems or develop policy.

4.3 FROM PROVISIONAL ISSUE TO SCIENTIFIC PROBLEM

4.3.1 Problems which are discarded

Once a provisional issue has been formulated, it can be developed further and converted into a definitive problem. It should not be forgotten however that some valid provisional issues are not developed but are discarded at this stage. These are not found in the literature. Apart from reasons which are linked to the strength and dominance of the current paradigm, as described in Chapter 1, a number of other reasons for this can be identified:

– the relevance of the issue at that time for the researcher. When the scope of a problem or its potential contribution to theory formulation is limited, an issue can have a low priority and be rejected;

– the status which can be derived from research results and the corresponding publicity value (consider for example the high publicity surrounding research in cold nuclear fusion, genetic engineering, etc.);

– limitation of finance for research. If costly research is not adequately funded, research questions may be dropped;

– suitability of the question for research. In practice, many issues have an obvious ethical facet. These questions not only concern the facts, but also have moral and social implications. Such questions are more suitable for discussion than for scientific research;

– the scope of the issue. Broad issues are often difficult to research. They may require restructuring into various subsections before being useful for research;

– ethical elements of the research process, for example experiments involving human beings;

– practical circumstances, such as:
  • time;
  • availability of experimental subjects;
  • necessary co-operation of others;
  • availability of structures and materials;
  • the lack of experience of the researcher.

4.3.2 Literature review

An initial question is usually not directly suitable for research. As was described in Chapter 2, further information gathered from a review of the literature is necessary before a general question can be converted into a scientific question. The literature available can be sub-divided into *conceptual* literature and *research* literature.

An important question in this context is: 'Where can the necessary literature be found?'

The most important sources are listed below.

1. In studying research and conceptual literature, the researcher will obviously find bibliographical information, which might merit further follow-up.

2. Bibliographies appear regularly listing the publications in a particular field which have appeared in a certain period. By searching for key words and/or author names, the researcher can glean much from those bibliographies.

3. Indexes are valuable. Whereas a bibliography usually refers to books, an index is concerned with articles which appeared during a particular period in a group of selected journals.

4. Abstracts provide short summaries of articles. Only a very small area of the field will be covered by this.

5. Book reviews, published in journals, are also an important source of information.

6. The consultation of specialists in a certain area may yield important literature references, certainly in the initial phase.

7. The 'computer search' is a very effective method for directed literature research. With the aid of key words, possibly in combination with logical search conditions, it is possible to obtain relevant information from international library files.

The contribution which can be made to an effective literature review by the support of effective library services and personnel cannot be overstated. A more detailed discussion of literature reviewing, which is an element of the research process in its own right, is presented in Chapter 5.

4.3.3 Definition of terms

From the literature review it is possible to proceed to defining the research question. This must be clearly formulated and embedded in a conceptual framework. The terms used in the question must be precisely defined.

Example

In the following illustration the effect of the patient's position in bed, varying from reclining to upright, upon central venous pressure (CVP) is investigated. The research is carried out among children who have undergone recent cardiac surgery. The objective is to find out whether the often troublesome and painful change of posture, which is considered necessary for CVP measuring, is actually needed. On the basis of the stated question the terms were formulated thus.

The use of central venous pressure (CVP) monitoring has been a long-standing practice with the pediatric population (Daily, 1985). Weesner, Rocchini & Rosenthal (1982) found that CVP monitoring was often all that was necessary in critically ill children. In children following cardiac surgery, accurate monitoring of right ventricular function, as reflected by the central venous or right atrial pressure, is crucial since right ventricular function and right heart anatomy are affected independently of left ventricular function and left heart anatomy.

An upright position results in changes in heart rate, stroke volume, and cardiac output by pooling of venous blood in the dependent extremities (Braunwald, 1984; Mohr, Smolinsky & Goor, 1982; Rapaport, Wong, Escobar & Marting, 1966). It has therefore been assumed that the supine position is necessary to achieve an accurate CVP reading. However, the supine position may be contraindicated in children following heart surgery due to increased intracranial pressure, respiratory compromise, or nasogastric feedings. Patient discomfort and sleep disruption may result from the hourly position change necessary to obtain CVP readings in the supine position. Additional nursing time is also required for frequent positioning of children. However, postural effects on CVP readings in children following cardiac surgery have not been examined. Thus this study examines the effect of backrest elevation on CVP readings in children, age 1 day to 9 years, following cardiac surgery.

The CVP reading was defined as the number in mmHg transmitted by a

Hewlett-Packard transducer and shown on the Hewlett-Packard monitor. If calibrated and zeroed in accordance with instruction in the *Hewlett-Packard Critical Care Network Operation Guide* (1982), the maximum error expected for the CVP readings is ± .1 per mmHg (S. Machacek, personal communication, April 15, 1987). Backrest elevation was defined as the degree of elevation of the child's stretcher or bed as measured by a protractor placed at the angle of the backrest. Two backrest elevations were examined, 0- and 30-degree.

L.B. Callow and B. Pieper (1989),
'Effect of backrest on central venous pressure in pediatric cardiac surgery',
in: *Nursing Research* 38/6, pp. 336-338

4.3.4 Hypotheses

Questions can have a general nature, especially when the extent of a phenomenon's occurrence is to be researched or when there are connections with other phenomena. This is the case with descriptive and exploratory investigations. When, however, explicit and exact predictions are formulated in a question, we call this a hypothesis. A hypothesis is a research question which fits into a particular programme of testing or *experimental research*. This programme takes place only after concrete predictions have been made on the basis of extensive theorising and earlier research (often of a descriptive and explorative nature).

A hypothesis is a statement which predicts the performance of a verifiable occurrence in certain conditions, based upon theoretical considerations. It is, therefore, suitable for research. The use of a hypothesis demonstrates that the research does *not* start from *coincidence*. In an experiment which tests a hypothesis, an attempt is made to verify something. The operative arrangement in the following example is that H_0 (the *null hypothesis*) is the hypothesis that nothing would change, while the alternative statement is formulated as in the H_1.

Example
Change of position is expected to reduce the occurrence of decubitus ulcers. The hypotheses used in research to test this might be stated as:
H_0: Change of position every two hours, in patients confined to bed, has no effect on the occurrence of decubitus ulcers.
H_1: Change of position every two hours, in patients confined to bed, reduces the occurrence of decubitus ulcers.

In the previous chapters it has become evident that in socio-scientific research, work can only be done in terms of probabilities, not of absolute statements and certainties. A hypothesis may present very concrete expectations. The results of experiments usually do not quite correspond to them. However, if the experimental results strongly tend towards one hypothesis or the other, this is normally a useful outcome.

Example
In testing the hypotheses above, concerning 'change of position and the occurrence of decubitus ulcers', the occurrence of superficial forms of skin blistering in one patient in an experimental group of 35 would not lead to doubt about the effect of the treatment. H_0 would still be dismissed.

However, when the difference between the null hypothesis and the research results gets bigger, the question arises as to whether that difference is due to chance factors or conditions in the research (related, for instance, to the representativeness of the sample group). It is possible to test whether deviations in the results are statistically insignificant, and do not suggest an inaccurate hypothesis. For this testing however, it is necessary to establish in advance how much risk there is of dismissing a hypothesis wrongly. The researcher does this by determining the level of significance, in advance, which will accurately test the hypotheses.

It may occur that a researcher, in very rare circumstances, dismisses an accurate zero hypothesis through miscalculating the significance of results. This is called a mistake of the first order. A mistake of the second order happens when an alternative hypothesis which is factually correct is not accepted, because the zero hypothesis is, wrongly, not dismissed. These first and second order mistakes, also known as Type I and Type II errors, are discussed at Chapter 9, section 9.3.2.

Four conditions should be met by a hypothesis.

1. It should be logically consistent. It must not predict results which are inherently contradictory;

2. A hypothesis should be stated as simply as possible;

3. The predictions deducible from a hypothesis must be verifiable. If they are not, the hypothesis cannot be tested;

4. A hypothesis must relate to a matter which can be clearly defined empirically. It should leave no doubt about what material is within its frame of reference.

4.4 THE DATA MATRIX

Each research question can be translated into the form of a data matrix. This is a useful method of breaking down research data unambiguously and ensuring its completeness. Through the matrix form it is made clear:

- which perceptual units one would like to contact, the perceptual unit being the empirical unit in which phenomena are to be perceived;

- which variables one would like to research (the variables are the characteristics to be measured in the perception units);

- which measuring procedures are to apply.

The matrix provides, as it were, the research question in a nutshell. It is the last stage of the reasoning process before the actual research. Thus the researcher who wants to investigate the hypothesis 'nurses can distinguish frightened patients from those who are less frightened' will be interested in the feelings of fear in, for example, cardiology patients. Among other things, the researcher will measure the variable 'fear'. People experience widely different degrees of fear, and some will score higher on the scale than others. The researcher will also have to record the nurses' assessment of each patient's fear. The attribution of a value on a scale to the variable 'fear' is called measurement in this example. This is the attribution of a single value to a variable within a well defined range. In this example, 'cardiology patients' constitutes the perceptual unit.

The above example makes up the data matrix shown in Figure 4.1:
- – variable 1: age
- – variable 2: sex
- – variable 3: fear
- – variable 4: etc

Perceptual unit	Variable 1	2	3	4	...	m
1	X_{11}	X_{12}	X_{13}	X_{14}	...	X_{1m}
2	X_{21}	X_{22}	X_{23}	X_{24}	...	.
3	X_{31}	X_{32}	X_{33}	X_{34}	...	.
.	.	.	.	.	...	.
.	.	.	.	.	...	.
.	.	.	.	.	...	.
n	X_{n1}	.	.	.	...	X_{nm}

Figure 4.1. The data matrix

Research unit
It is important to note that the perceptual unit and the research unit do not always need to be identical.

Example
In an investigation into the effects that different ways of organising nursing care have on patient satisfaction, the perceptual unit is the patient. The research unit, the thing about which you wish to make a statement, would in this case be the ward where nursing is organised in a particular way.

The phase of formulating the research question ends with the determination of the type of research that is going to be carried out. In general, the selection of the type of research depends on the question and its theoretical context (see Chapter 6 for a further discussion about the different types of research).

STUDY ACTIVITY 2
Take three issues as you formulated them in the first study activity of this chapter. Convert them into research questions. Indicate in each case which research units are to be used, which variables you are going to measure and which perceptual units you will work with.

4.5 SUMMARY
This chapter looked at the research question or research problem. The research question is generally seen as the guiding principle which gives direction to the

research. Three source areas for questions were described: professional practice, the testing of theories and research assignments.

A fundamental step in the conversion of a global question into one suitable for research is a study of the literature, for which different methods were described. Attention was given to reasons why global questions may not always be developed into research questions.

Issues relating to the hypothesis and the role of research in verifying it, and to the data matrix as an aid to encapsulating all elements of the research question, were then addressed.

5

THE LITERATURE REVIEW: PERSPECTIVES AND METHODS

5.1 APPROACHES

It is generally expected that a report of a research project should include a review of the literature, either within the introduction or as a separate section. Such reviews vary considerably in style, depth and content. However the review in a thesis is expected to be much more comprehensive than, for example, the type of brief review commonly found in papers in learned journals.

Many research reports appear to adopt a scatter-gun strategy whereby a very large number of references are quoted without any real attempt to analyse or critique. Others briefly quote a smaller number of references, with varying depths of analysis, but do not present a comprehensive review of the subject or field. A review which simply lists references or which omits significant contributions in the existing literature on a topic cannot be considered satisfactory.

In essence there is here a dilemma of depth versus breadth. If the scope is too broad and an attempt is made to encompass the whole available literature, it is virtually impossible for the researcher to analyse and critique in depth. Embarking on such a marathon task can greatly extend the duration of the project or alternatively seriously limit the time available for work on other parts of the project. Alternatively, if detailed in-depth 'critiquing' of each reference quoted is undertaken, it is probably impossible to cover all the really significant contributions which should have been referenced without running into similar problems of timing and balance.

There is significant pressure on researchers to go beyond simply listing references in the review. Lack of adequate critiquing is clearly seen as a cardinal sin, probably because it is the sin most frequently committed! For example, Best (1970) advises that:
'In searching related literature the researcher should note important elements:
(a) Reported problems or closely related problems that have been investigated.
(b) Design of the study, including procedures employed and data-gathering instruments used.
(c) Populations that were studied.
(d) Variables that could have affected the findings.
(e) Pitfalls or faults that were apparent.
(f) Recommendations for further research'. (p.29)

There can be little doubt that these elements are important in terms of evaluating research literature and ascertaining its importance to a particular research project. However, to attempt to include detailed reporting of such critical analysis for each reference cited would be a daunting task. Indeed Kidder (1981) stresses the need to be brief, to only present pertinent points and to condense as much as possible without sacrificing clarity.

5.2 FUNCTIONS OF A LITERATURE REVIEW

There are four main functions of a literature review. These are:

1. To give reasons why the topic is of sufficient importance for it to be researched. For example, for a study on the 'smoking behaviour of people with peripheral vascular disease', literature on the health implications for the individual and the economic costs of treatment could be cited in support of the project.

2. To provide the reader with a brief up-to-date account and discussion of literature on the issues relevant to the topic. For a study on the 'learning styles of student nurses', the review could include the following:
(a) a brief account of the development of learning styles in nurse education. If this is not a historical study this section should only aim to give the reader an account of how, and if, learning styles in nurse education have evolved;
(b) a brief discussion of the main learning styles;
(c) the policies and views of relevant bodies, eg, the National Boards for Nursing, Midwifery and Health Visiting or the Royal College of Nursing, on learning styles;
(d) the views of the experts in the field as reflected in text books and journals.

3. To provide a conceptual and theoretical context in which the topic for research can be situated. For example in a study on 'non-compliance with medical advice' some of the literature on health belief theories such as the Health Belief model, the Reasoned Action model and the Social Learning Theory would provide the backdrop against which the topic and the relevant issues could be discussed. The operational definition of concepts is often facilitated by reviewing how others have attempted this particular task. In the above example it is useful to find out how 'compliance' is operationally defined in the conceptual as well as in the research literature.

4. To discuss relevant research carried out on the same topic or similar topics (if no previous research has been carried out on the proposed topic). This does not mean that a full critique of every research project is required. The skill of the researcher in including the relevant aspects of these studies as well as his/her ability to be critical and draw conclusions is particularly important. This critique of other similar research projects can be presented in a number of ways. Some researchers include a section in the literature review chapter solely devoted to research projects on the topic. Others refer to these projects as the need arises in the review.

STUDY ACTIVITY 1

Go to your library and do literature searches on health belief theories:
a. the Health Belief model;
b. the Reasoned Action model;
c. Social Learning Theory.
Write a brief description of each, quoting the references you consulted.

Sometimes a research report has no separate chapter on literature review. Instead, the relevant literature is integrated in the text as the need arises. Thus in chapters where research designs, data collection and analysis, and conclusions are presented, the relevant literature is reviewed. It is argued that for reasons of impact and ease of reading, and because of practicalities such as fieldwork-initiated returns to the literature, this is an appropriate approach in many instances, particularly in qualitative research.

A useful way to summarise research projects is in a tabular form (Figure 5.1). By grouping research under these headings the similarities, differences and contradictions will be more obvious. Such a table provides valuable information at a glance.

5.3 FOCUS AND APPROACH

The issue of relevance is of the highest importance. The onus is on the researcher to seek out and review material which has relevance to his/her project. Where literature is highly and directly relevant it should be analysed in detail, its strengths and weaknesses identified, and the relevance to current research explicitly rather than implicitly illustrated (Burns and Grove, 1987). However many examples, in unpublished theses (eg, Sellick, 1977; Reid, 1983), and in published monographs (eg, Gallego, 1983; Paykel and Griffith, 1983) quote some references as supporting sources without analysing or even describing the source. This would seem to be reasonable if set in a context within which important sources are closely examined while others are presented as additional corroborative evidence.

The usual approach encountered is, as indicated above, that which presents a self-contained section reviewing the literature in the opening stages of the report. This is particularly the case in quantitative research, where the review is usually intended to establish the state of knowledge relating to the research area, and by so doing establish the jump-off point for extending this knowledge.

With the exception of variations in depth and breadth of analysis and operational definitions of relevance implicit in choice of references, the pattern is more or less standard. And it is of course the pattern advocated in most standard texts and papers on research methodology, eg, Parahoo and Reid (1988), Burns and Grove (op. cit.), Verhonick and Seaman (1978), Best (op. cit.).

Figure 5.1 Tabulation of literature reviewed

Title of Project	Year	Approach (Qualitative/ Quantitative)	Sample and Sampling Method	Methods	Findings

Some researchers do, however, employ different approaches. For example, in historical research, literature reviewed may in itself be the data under investigation. In
other instances, such as in qualitative social research, the review may be used to
compare with, or extend and elaborate upon, research findings. In such instances the
common approach described above may be deliberately avoided. In this context
Oiler (1982) suggests that the review should be left until the end of the project, so that
the opinions, conclusions, etc, of others to be found in the literature do not create
researcher bias from the outset. In similar vein Chinn (1985) writes of the 'myth of
higher authority' perpetuated by commencing scholarly works with a review of
'authoritative' literature. She suggests that:

> 'The halo effect that an idea or belief acquires by being published is a remarkable
> transition that I can only perceive as being magic'. (p.48)

While not completely rejecting the positivistic science paradigm, Chinn suggests that
nursing knowledge may benefit from moving from an exclusively 're-search' model
to one which adopts a 'future search' perspective. Drawing on the ideas of Heide
(1982), she suggests that this might include debunking the myths of scientific
enterprise by questioning not only the unquestioning acceptance of available literature as legitimate and 'true', but also the supremacy of the scientific method in the
quest for truth.

Much qualitative research also presents literature review throughout the report. For
example, Fontana (1977), in a study of elderly people in a nursing home, conducted
from an essentially phenomenological perspective, completely integrates literature
review with data collection and analysis throughout his report. In studies such as this
the approach is clearly appropriate, for it allows comparison, illustration and
elaboration at the points of highest impact for the reader. There are also practical

reasons for this approach. Often in such research it is the data-rich field notes which direct the researcher back to the literature again and again as new questions and problems arise. Indeed Kidder (op. cit.) identifies such movement back and forth between field work and the literature as being the most common pattern in practice.

STUDY ACTIVITY 2
List three advantages each for:
a. a literature review presented as a separate, discrete section or chapter of the research report;
b. a literature review which is integrated throughout the research report rather than as a separate section or chapter.

5.4 PRINCIPLES
Running through the literature on review methodology can be found a number of important principles. In most instances the principles which should be adopted for guiding the review of literature are as follows:

5.4.1 Relevance
Probably that which is paramount among these is the principle of relevance. Batey (1977) suggests that sources referred to should only be those which are pertinent to the research project and which provide related knowledge. This should be the first test of choice for references included in any study.

5.4.2 Depth
The need to ensure that sources are adequately described, analysed and 'critiqued' has already been emphasised above. This principle should be applied particularly to those sources which are considered to be highly and directly relevant to the research project. Other sources, considered to be of less vital relevance are quoted to support points of view. In these situations a judgement is made, in the context of limited time and resources, not to conduct in-depth critiques.

5.4.3 Breadth
The principle of selecting highly relevant sources for more comprehensive examination must be partnered by a principle of attempting to ensure that *all relevant* contributions to the literature are examined. This principle may be applied in two senses. Firstly, as indicated above, while some highly important sources are discussed in detail others are also included albeit at a less detailed level of analysis. Secondly, the review is not necessarily limited to empirical research, but may also draw from theoretical, philosophical and (in the case of health care research) clinical literature.

There is often a danger, particulary within the newer professions such as nursing, to strive for scientific respectability to the extent that non-empirical knowledge is held in disdain. However, it is important to recognise that theoretical literature points to the stage of knowledge development in terms of the accumulated body of research information and scholarly thinking. The same type of argument can hold for literature which is essentially philosophical, or indeed literature which reflects the professional or clinical judgement of acknowledged experts. It is important, nevertheless, to be selective in including such literature. Kidder (op. cit.) cautions against including literature which merely reflects opinions or beliefs which are not based on empirical evidence or careful analysis.

A literature search should span the range of written sources such as textbooks, articles, newspaper material, policy documents, research theses, censuses and survey reports, etc. However, an over-representation of textbooks at the expense of articles from learned journals is likely to indicate that the search is too narrow. Articles tend to be more up-to-date on topical issues than text books. A reliance on anecdotes or articles from the popular press would not be desirable as these would contribute little to the academic status of the review.

Another indication of a poor literature review is when most of the references come from only one or two journals or textbooks. Some nursing research topics clearly require researchers to consult not only nursing but also non-nursing sources. References to books and journals in the fields of psychology, sociology and medicine would indicate the breadth of the literature search. Although it may not be possible to consult all the literature published, it is important to avoid an ethnocentric bias, by referring to relevant literature from other countries as well.

Finally, a list of references gives an indication of the author's use of primary and secondary sources. Primary sources are original documents, eg, original research reports or papers in learned journals which report research. Secondary sources are not the original documents but reports or references to these, usually made by others; in essence such references, while they may be highly relevant and valuable, must be recognised as second-hand information. Primary sources are preferred whenever possible, since it allows the researcher to give his or her own interpretation of the original work instead of seeing it through the eyes of other authors.

Overall, a list of references can provide valuable insight on the breadth of the literature search. A balanced tilted towards up-to-date references to articles from various learned journals, from various disciplines and not reflecting an ethnocentric bias would usually be indicative of a comprehensive literature review.

5.4.4 Honest presentation

In most research areas there is some literature of relevance to be found. Indeed more often than not, there are vast quantities of literature which can be adjudged as relevant, particularly if a fairly open definition of relevance is being employed. In such circumstances it is possible to quote large numbers of references without the researcher actually having read them in detail, if at all! Indeed the researcher could be in a position to select only literature which fits in with his world view or which shows his own research in its best light. Gunter (1981) sees within this situation a fundamental ethical problem, for deliberately presenting a biased review can only be viewed as a breach of ethics.

An important principle is that of consciously including only literature which had been carefully studied and which was honestly considered to be of relevance. In addition, honest attempts must be made to present a balanced review. That is, to present literature which as a body of references accurately reflects the available knowledge as opposed to presenting only that which fits in with the researcher's beliefs and assumptions.

STUDY ACTIVITY 3

Select a paper presenting a research report in any of the nursing journals contained in your college/university library. Read the report, paying particular attention to the literature review. Write a criticism of the literature review, with at least 200 words each on relevance, depth, breadth and honest presentation. You may find it helpful to ask a fellow student or your supervisor to comment on your analysis.

5.5 FRAMEWORK AND SYNTHESIS

The review of literature should be an integral and important part of the research report. It is sometimes the case that researchers consider the review as the soft part of the project. In their anxiety to proceed to what is viewed as the really important work - data collection and analysis - this aspect is glossed over. Indeed in some cases the review gives the impression of having been grafted onto the report, of having been rushed through without much real thought given to structure and relationship to the research design. This is essentially a regrettable and misguided approach. The review is an important and essential element of research. Doing the review is as much 'doing' research as is any other stage of the research process, and its importance should be recognised in this context.

In any research project an attempt must be made to recognise this importance, and to ensure that the review is integrated into the overall research framework. As suggested earlier the review of literature may be related to, and integrated with, the overall framework in two ways. In the first approach, a general review of the literature pertaining to the overall field of study is included, usually as a separate chapter or section of the research report. The second approach involves an integration of commentary on the literature reviewed throughout the research report.

The decision to adopt the first or second approach, or indeed a combination of the two, is a matter for the researcher. The important things to remember are that this decision in itself reflects an important research question, and that the literature review is an important part of the overall research project. As such it must be submitted to the same standards of critical analysis and ethical concern as other parts of the research project.

STUDY ACTIVITIES

4. A nurse wants to research the job satisfaction of qualified nurses working with elderly mentally ill people in hospitals. List the issues which you think should be discussed in the literature review.

5. Select a research article from a learned nursing journal and comment on the following:

a. the balance of references to journal articles in relation textbooks;

b. reference to non-nursing sources;

c. the use of primary sources and secondary sources;

d. the presence or absence of ethnocentric bias in the list of references.

5.6 SUMMARY

This chapter stressed that the literature review is a vital and essential aspect of the research process. Reviewing the literature, it is argued, is not a grafted on 'extra', or unimportant aspect of the final report, but is in fact an element of *doing* research. It is suggested that the four main functions of a literature review are: to indicate the importance of the proposed research; to provide an up-to-date account of relevant issues; to provide a conceptual and theoretical context; and, to present an account of relevant research on the same or similar topics. The review may be presented as a separate section or chapter of the research report. Alternatively, it may be integrated throughout the report, with literature pertinent to a particular aspect, eg, research design, data collection or analysis, being review when that aspect is being addressed. Irrespective of the style, the reviewer must address principles of relevance, depth, breadth and honest presentation. It is particularly important that where possible primary sources which report on research relevant to the study are included. As an important aspect of the research process, the literature review must be submitted to the same standards of critical analysis and ethical concern as for other aspects of the research process.

6

RESEARCH TYPES, RESEARCH DESIGN AND RESEARCH STRATEGY

6.1 INTRODUCTION

After the formulation of the question and its theoretical context, and after the literature has been at least initially reviewed, the researcher comes to the question: 'Which research design corresponds best to the problem?' In a small number of cases this research design is dictated by the nature of the research. For example, in an investigation into the efficacy of drugs, neither the patient nor the observer must know who receives the medicine and who the placebo ('double blind research'). Usually, however, the researcher has a choice. Which option is chosen will depend largely on the relationship between the theoretical framework, the formulated problem and the practical possibilities open to the researcher. An illustration of this is given in the following example.

Example
In carrying out nursing duties in an old people's home, a student becomes particularly interested in the subject of urinary incontinence among the elderly. On the basis of this interest a provisional problem is formulated: does residence in an institution, like a residential home, contribute to the occurrence of urinary incontinence?
Evidence from background reading indicates that there is further room for exploration of the field and scope for theory formation about the environmental factors which may contribute to the occurrence of incontinence. The question is therefore reformulated: to what extent does urinary incontinence occur among elderly patients in various domestic and institutional situations?

Obviously, if the patterns of occurrence of a phenomenon have not yet been recorded, no research can be done on the factors which might explain these patterns. Finding and recording the occurrences must be the first step in the research. On the other hand, if some provisional work has been done this will help to focus the research, pushing it towards, for example, the verification of a hypothesis. This shows, once again, the value of a thorough and extensive review of the literature.
In the following example, it can be seen how the practical circumstances of the research have an impact on the research design.

Example
A researcher who is interested in the experiences of parents visiting children in paediatric wards can develop this issue in various ways, depending largely on how far the parents can be expected to participate.
1. A limited sample of 15 parent couples can be selected and asked about their

experiences immediately after their visit, in an open or semi-structured interview.

2. A structured questionnaire can be sent to 100 parent couples, selected from the hospital files, with a request to complete and return them.

3. Information about the experience of the parents can be obtained by means of participant observations during visiting over a defined period.

In the example, three different research plans are outlined, and each will yield information about the issue. But it should be noted that the chosen research form partly determines the conclusions which may later be drawn from the research.
In the choice of research design, there is a tension between methodological demands and considerations on the one hand and the practical feasibility of the procedures on the other.

STUDY ACTIVITY 1
In Chapter 4, Study Activity 2 you formulated three research questions. For each one develop three different general ways of collecting the information you would need in order to answer these questions.

6.2 RESEARCH TYPES
Essentially, three basic forms of research can be distinguished.

6.2.1 Descriptive research
This type of research sets out to describe a phenomenon systematically and to organise it into a useful structure. The survey carried out during a National Census is a clear example of descriptive research.
A theoretical framework is useful here. For example, describing a nursing home population in terms of Orem's self-care theory helps to establish a structure for the descriptions. Often, however, the conceptual structure is missing in descriptive research, so that interpretations and explanations become rather arbitrary. One characteristic of good descriptive research is the explicit statement of structure according to which the research is done. The significance of descriptive research should not be neglected; good and extensive descriptive research is the foundation of valid follow-up work.

6.2.2 Exploratory research
The objective of exploratory research is the development of a general theory and the formation and selection of hypotheses. Here, the researcher starts from a theoretical framework which is not yet complete. Such a framework might arise from the results of descriptive research into a nursing problem. Through exploratory research, attempts are made to find connections between different sets of results. Empirical trends and patterns can be looked for and stated. These connections and patterns should then lead to the formation of a theory and of verifiable hypotheses. Good exploratory research should deal with plenty of material with a high information content. The examination of this material demands a lot of the researcher; theories and hypotheses

from different presuppositions and angles should be developed all the time, without actually testing and establishing the underlying theoretical principle.

6.2.3 Verifying research

Verifying research is, or rather appears to be, the last phase in the process, in which the developed theory is tested. Verifying research does not constitute the end point of the empirical cycle, which should be thought of rather more as a spiral, where the solution of one question leads to the immediate emergence of others. The area in which verifying research takes place is not reality, but theory. This means that one does not strive for an abundance and richness of research data, as one does in descriptive and exploratory research, but for unequivocal findings, which allow convincing theories to be established. In verifying research an attempt is made to explain the effect of one or more factors on a situation. Thus the causal relation between phenomena might be shown. Hypotheses are developed which make concrete predictions about what will happen in certain situations. These hypotheses can be dismissed or verified.

The three research types described here are ideal types (i.e. representations with all the characteristics of the types, which seldom if ever occur in reality). In practice, hybrids of the various types are possible within one research design.

6.3 CHOICE OF RESEARCH DESIGN

Apart from the research type, which is determined by the nature of the problem and the theoretical context, several other issues affect the actual execution of the research. The researcher can collect data in various ways, starting from the same research question but using different instruments or different groups of test subjects.

These choices relate to different research designs. The research design is a blueprint which takes into account considerations such as:
  – *the size of the random sample in relation to the target population*. Obviously, when a researcher presents findings about the opinion of the British general public on, say, religious affairs, a larger random group will be needed than when the research is confined to the opinions of churchgoers in a certain part of a town;
  – *the number and the nature of the variables which are researched*. Here too it will be plain that in the case of an exploratory inquiry within a large random sample, the number of variables will probably be greater than in the case of a small one;
  – *the time available and the methods of data collection to be used*.
The considerations which can underlie these choices will discussed in later chapters.

STUDY ACTIVITY 2

Study the following extract from a research publication and describe the research type and the research design used.

This research study was established to examine the relationship between the use of coping strategies and burnout among a group of staff nurses. The approach taken was that nurses who would experience burnout used strategies of avoidance, self control and confrontation. Those who would experience lower levels of burnout would use problem solving approaches, positive re-appraisal and sought social support.

Method of research
500 nurses in four hospitals were contacted following a meeting with a nursing administrator in each hospital. The contact took the form of a package which contained a covering letter explaining that confidentiality would be assured along with forms for completion. One month after distribution 150 completed questionnaires were returned, a response rate of 30%.

The questionnaires
The instrument took the form of the Maslach Burnout Inventory containing 25 items measuring three dimensions of burnout – namely emotional exhaustion, depersonalization and personal accomplishment. The subscales contained items which measured such things as fatigue, unfeeling and impersonal attitude to clients and feelings of competence.

The Ways of Coping Scale was an instrument which contained 66 items examining eight modes of coping. The responses were categorized using a Likert scale.

The scores achieved on the burnout inventory were as follows:

Dimension	Mean Score	Expected Range
Emotional exhaustion	20.4	18-29
Depersonalization	6.37	6-11
Personal accomplishment	35.3	34-39

S.B. Ceslowitz (1989),
Burnout and coping strategies among hospital staff nurses,
Journal of Advanced Nursing, 14, pp. 553-557

The research design is built onto the question and the research type, with methodological considerations determining to a large degree the decisions that are taken.

6.4 RESEARCH STRATEGY

Following decisions about the research type and design, the research strategy is developed. Considerations about both the research design and the research strategy tend to be looked at together however, and the difference between them is not as easy to distinguish as suggested here.

The research strategy entails further development of the research design. One important consideration is the procedure to be followed during the research. The strategy can be defined as a more or less standard combination of methods, techniques and procedures. It is, as it were, a basic pattern of research, embedded in the questions, the research type and the design. A number of important strategies are discussed below.

6.4.1 Study of source material

The study of source material concentrates in general on written material and is used when an answer is thought to be available in the literature. Attention is usually focused on a limited number of variables and the number of perceptual units included is limited partly because the study of source material is rather labour intensive. This strategy offers reasonable control possibilities, since the research stages can be checked through afterwards. Two main approaches can be distinguished: content analysis and source criticism.

1. Content analysis

Content analysis is a method of categorising verbal data. This is very labour intensive, but has the advantage that there are possibilities for correction later in the research. Large demands are made on the researcher's creativity. The source material may be on tape or already typed out verbatim. It can be analysed for its literal contents, its emotional tone and its intentions.

Example
A researcher is particularly interested in the attitude of the media to campaigns by nurses for better working conditions. It is decided to subject the coverage by a number of authoritative media to content analysis. News tapes, tapes of current affairs programmes and newspaper articles are analysed.

In content analysis, use of pilot studies is recommended for testing and readjusting the categories that will be used to assess and structure the findings.

2. Source criticism

An important problem researchers face in source material is: Which points can be accepted from a document and which should be dismissed? Source criticism, which is often used in historical studies, deals with the reliability of sources of all kinds including papers, books, pamphlets and scientific studies. A number of relevant questions within source criticism are:
- under what circumstances was the data collected and how does this affect the reliability?
- were the methods and instruments used to collect the data adequate?
- how established is the expertise and objectivity of the person who collected the data?
- to what extent is the terminology clear and unambiguous?

Example
A researcher wants to compare the concepts, visions and theories of nursing in the USA with those in the UK. In order to make a valid comparison, a number of standard nursing texts which are used in nursing colleges are analysed.

It will be clear that reliable source criticism is more difficult than it seems at first.

6.4.2 Field work

Field work usually involves qualitative research into the social structures of communities, with the researcher working within the area to be studied, participating in the life and social system of that area. This form of research is particularly suited to questions about social processes which specifically concern one particular group or for which only one group is available for study. In addition, the field study offers the advantage that behaviour may be observed 24 hours a day, so that it can be interpreted and reinterpreted during this period and can be tested more than once. There is no need to wait for the data to be complete before processing, analysis and interpretation can be started.

Field work is eminently suitable for exploratory research projects where theory formulation is a more important aim than the finding of causal explanatory models. This strategy is often used in cultural anthropology and sociology. The possibilities for control are limited.

6.4.3 Case study

A case study is research dealing with one individual case, for instance, the care problems of a school pupil suffering from disturbed behaviour. This research form is a type of field research, restricted to a single individual or a small social system. Establishing the reliability of data derived from case studies is problematic.

Researchers doing field work or carrying out case studies use a number of theoretical approaches to the collection and analysis of data. Among the most commonly used are phenomenology and symbolic interactionism. These are fully discussed in Chapter 3.

6.4.4 Survey

The survey is a large-scale investigation into occurrences or the connections between them. This is a form of exploratory research, of a strongly quantitative nature. It focuses on directly perceptible phenomena, with the data acquired being processed statistically. The survey concentrates on everyday life, not on the artificially created situation that might be used in an experiment. A great deal of socio-scientific research is done through the survey.

The survey can be characterised as:

– easily applicable to large groups of respondents – for example, suitable for spot random sampling of a population on a large scale. (Groups to be spot checked should be selected carefully, because conclusions may be applied to the whole population);

– exploratory, suitable for a broad introductory approach;

– based on relatively open questions, mostly directed at describing population characteristics or defining and establishing connections between variables. These variables are often grouped around a central theme;

– designed to be based on a genuine random sample.

There are many specialised terms used in research reports and literature in connection with surveys. Some of these are outlined here.

– Multi random indication (see also cohort-study below): research can be made in a number of random samplings.

– Transverse, cross-sectional: studies are made simultaneously of two groups differing in, say, age or development so as to be able to establish the changes across time. It is a simpler and less expensive form of research, with quicker results, than a cohort-study.

– Cohort-study: a group composed at random is followed over a relatively long period of time and regular measurements are carried out among random samples from the group. This is especially useful in education, for instance to follow a group of primary school-leavers during their further school careers. (This is referred to as prospective research).

– Longitudinal: the opposite of cross-sectional research; data is collected at several points in time over a defined period.

6.4.5 The experiment

The experiment is empirical research which examines the connection between variables. Attention focuses on the effect that altering one variable has upon another. The variable which is controlled by the researcher is called the *independent* variable. The other, in which the effect is measured, is called the *dependent* variable.
Examples of experimental questions are:

– what is the effect of information and instruction on the post-operative recovery of the patient?

– what is the effect of medicine A on sleeping rhythm?

A fundamental precondition for experimental research is that factors which might affect the results should be kept under control. This can be achieved by ensuring that the effects of these factors are known, or by working with two groups which differ only in one independent factor. If there are factors whose impact is known, it must be ensured that they occur in equal frequency across both groups.
If an experiment is to be valid, observations should be made among the experimental group receiving treatment and also among a control group not receiving the treatment. A subject should have equal chances of ending up in the experimental or the control group. For example, in an experiment on the effect of leadership on study achievements, sex can be an important factor. The researcher will therefore match the subjects in couples and will then allocate each couple to one group or the other. In other situations subjects may be formed into pairs who share the same characteristics. One of the pair is then allocated to the experimental group and the other to the control group.
In a laboratory experiment the subjects are invited to come to the laboratory to participate. A field experiment takes place in the subject's natural surroundings. In the laboratory , disturbing influences which might affect the outcome can be kept under control, while this is not the case in the field. However, the artificiality of the laboratory can often be a drawback.

Example
A classic example of laboratory experiment using an original plan is the Milgram research (see Milgram, 1963; 1964). Milgram used 'stooges' in his experiment. The real subjects were individuals asked to assist in what they were told was an experiment which involved the teaching of word pairs. These 'assistants' were not aware that they were teaching the word pairs to experimental subjects who were stooges in collusion with the researcher. The assistants (real subjects) had seen the stooges at the beginning of the research tied to a chair. Thereafter assistants and stooges sat in separate rooms, communicating by an intercom. If the stooge gave an incorrect answer or no answer, the real subject was to punish him/her by administering an electric shock. The shock increased in voltage each time. It had been explained to the real subject that some shocks could be very painful and even lethal. (Obviously this was not actually true.)
Despite the pleading and begging to stop the electric shocks and the expressions of pain or even the silences which followed their administration, about 60% of the actual subjects continued inflicting shocks which, had they been real, might have proved lethal. In the case of refusal or hesitation by the subject the experiment leader simply said: 'Please carry on, the experiment requires you to continue'. The purpose of Milgram's experiment was to measure the degree of compliance to authority.

Basic plan of the experiment
To demonstrate the basic plan of an experiment, the following example will be useful. A research study is established to find out whether direct information supplied prior to surgery affects the experience of fear among children. (This example is fictitious, and ignores the ethical aspects of not supplying such information.)
This information which is supplied gives an explanation of everything that is going to happen in the pre-operative phase, a limited explanation about the operative surgery itself and an explanation about what the children may expect in the post-operative phase. It is offered at a level of understanding suited to the child's age. The experience of fear is measured with two specially designed instruments: a questionnaire and an observation scale.
The experimental plan is called 'pre-test post-test design'. The experimental and control groups are composed in such a way that there is no chance of differences between them affecting the results. The variable being influenced – in this case 'fear' – is called the *dependent variable*, while the variable which influences it – in this case 'information' – is called the *independent variable*. Thus, in all experiments, the manipulated independent variable is the *cause* and the changing dependent variable is the *effect*. This of course assumes that the cause leads to an expected effect and allows us to discuss the null hypothesis. In some cases there is no significant change in the dependent variable, or it changes in an unexpected direction.

Before the experimental treatment begins, initial measurement of the level of the children's fear should take place. Then the explanations described above are given only to the 'experimental group' children.If a difference in fear level between the experimental and the control group is found in post-test measurement, this difference can be attributed to the experimental treatment since this is the only character-istic in which the two groups differ.

However, initial measuring can have an educative effect or a disturbing impact on the subjects. In the example above, the fear of the children might be increased by the advance measuring. To gauge the effect of advance measuring, the researcher can opt for a comparable third and fourth group without advance measurement, with group 3 undergoing the experimental treatment and the post-test measurement afterwards and group 4 only undergoing the final measurement. The comparison of the post-test measurements between the four groups makes it possible to distinguish the effects of advance measuring and the effect of the experimental treatment. This test plan is represented in figure 6.1. This is often referred to as the Solomon Four-Group Design, after its original designer.

	Pre- Test		Post- Test	
group 1: R	O	X	O	experimental group
group 2: R	O		O	control group
group 3: R		X	O	
group 4: R			O	

R: at random appointment
O: observation and measuring
X: experimental treatment, in this case information supply

Figure 6.1 Four-group experimental design

However, it is not always possible to carry out initial measurement. In the above example, for instance, it might be very awkward to organise two separate measurements of fear. The children in the research would be able to recognise the questionnaire the second time and would, therefore, not give reliable answers. The researcher has to ensure that initial testing does not give rise to foreknowledge. The advance measurement should use another, comparable, instrument. If such instru-ments are not available, the researcher might make do with a 'post-test-only design'. Because of the random allocation it can be assumed that differences between children themselves, regarding the pre-operative fear, are divided equally among the groups. We have seen that the experiment is directed at establishing causal connections, with the number of variables and the number of perceptual units being limited. The control opportunities are great, especially in the case of the laboratory experiment.

6.5 SUMMARY
The following research types have been discussed in this chapter; descriptive, exploratory and experimental research. These research types have been shown to be basic classes. The research design is, as it were, the blueprint for the carrying out of the research. The design follows on from the question. The research strategy then provides for further development of the research procedure. Within the strategy the methods and techniques of the research are chosen. Descriptions were given of the strategies of source study, field study, case study, the survey and the experiment.

7

THE COLLECTION OF DATA

7.1 INTRODUCTION

Nursing and paramedical research is empirical, so in carrying it out, data must be collected empirically. This chapter looks at how the actual research takes place and how variables are assessed and measured. It examines how data are collected and considers the sources from which it originates. It investigates direct and indirect data collection, and the three basic collection techniques of observation, questioning and measuring.

7.2 DATA SOURCES

Data can be collected directly or indirectly.

7.2.1 Indirect data sources

Indirect data is information which has been collected by other institutions and researchers. It has the important advantage of being available and accessible. This reduces the time and cost of data collection considerably. A researcher using indirect sources is dependent on the way the work was originally done, however, and this can be a disadvantage. Three kinds of indirect sources may be noted.

1. *Official statistical material.* Data are collected by several institutions. As well as the well-known Office of Population and Census Surveys (OPCS), which operates on a national level, regional and local authorities and institutions also collect information. These include Regional and District Councils, Health Authorities, Chambers of Commerce, consultancies, job centres, training agencies, etc. The material they collect is normally made available for research; however, the researcher may not be aware of the existence or extent of these databanks, or may not know where to find them.

Official statistical material can be very useful in, for example, research into the occurrence of demographic phenomena, road safety, etc.

STUDY ACTIVITY 1

Investigate the demographic structure of the population in your home town. Make use of official statistical material.

There are a number of possible drawbacks to the use of official sources. These include the manner and the time in which the data were collected and recorded. Collection is often annual, whereas the researcher may prefer to have material recorded every quarter, for instance. The data might relate to populations which do not correspond with those that the researcher is investigating, or it may have been structured in an unsuitable way.

2. *Scientific publications.* The significance of thorough background reading of specialist literature has already been stressed in Chapter 5. While this may not make research entirely unnecessary, it may reduce the amount of work to be done.

3. *Data files from past research.* Databanks have been created from the results in large scale research, especially that commissioned by offical bodies. These are generally available for further analysis or as a control for new research.

7.2.2 Direct data sources

Direct data is derived from the researcher's own perceptions. The following sources may be noted.

1. Recorded material and inanimate objects. All of the documents which society produces may be studied. This includes not only legislation, magazines, papers, films, radio and TV broadcasts and archive material news, but also pamphlets, graffiti, etc. Within a hospital, annual reports, reports of nursing wards, conference minutes, sick lists and the like could be examined. Objects which might provide data can range from clothing to surgical instruments.

The extent to which the resuscitation trolley has been tidied up might be investigated, as might the amount and nature of food left-overs which are sent back to the kitchen.

2. Spontaneous verbal and non-verbal behaviour. Spontaneous behaviour is that which happens in natural situations, when an experiment is not taking place. Non-verbal behaviour includes, for example, the time taken for nurses to react to a patient buzzer, or the places taken by the participants in a meeting in relation to each other. An obvious example of verbal behaviour is use of jargon among certain professional groups. The different ways in which nurses talk about patients in different settings such as a psychiatric hospital, a general hospital, a hospital for people who have a learning disability, or a nursing home is interesting.

In general, research into spontaneous behaviour is labour-intensive, because it is difficult to predict when useful behaviour patterns will occur.

3. Induced behaviour, with or without the foreknowledge of the subject. Researchers usually do not observe behaviour passively. Usually, reactions are induced and then examined. The great benefit is that the researcher does not have to wait until the behaviour occurs spontaneously. This is an efficient procedure, but it can never be known for certain that the induced behaviour is the same as the spontaneous behaviour would have been.

This problem emerges particularly in situations where the subjects have been told that they are under observation. If nurses on a ward know their approach to patients of differing ethnic origins is being investigated, it is very likely that little difference will be found.

Other considerations include the ethics of certain working procedures, for example, recording behaviour with a hidden camera, or telling the subject that the question is different from the one actually being investigated (this is what happened in the Milgram experiment, discussed in Section 6.4.5).

Example
A classic experiment is the Asch experiment (1952). Responses were induced without the subject knowing exactly what the experiment entailed. The subjects were shown a line drawn on a chart then asked to select from three lines drawn on a different chart the line which corresponded most closely in length with the line on the first chart. However, in each group of eight 'subjects', there was one actual subject and seven accomplices (stooges) of the test leader who had been told to give identical but erroneous answers. The objective of the research was to investigate the reaction of the subject to being the only one giving correct answers. In fact, about 30% of the real subjects gave the same erroneous answer as the other group members, despite the fact that the mistakes were glaringly obvious.

7.3 TECHNIQUES FOR DATA COLLECTION

7.3.1 *Observation*

Observation, in principle, consists of observing phenomena in order to gain insight into how and why they happen.

The term 'observation', if interpreted freely, includes all research. In the more strict sense used here, it means the direct or indirect observation by a human observer of a phenomenon in order to be able to describe it and help to contribute to its understanding. The observer tries to influence the phenomenon as little as possible. A number of points can be made about observation:

- it is based on real events; it is actual behaviour that is observed, not verbal responses as in a questionnaire;
- it is a rather labour-intensive method;
- the processing and interpretation of the acquired material is difficult.

Observation is used especially in descriptive and exploratory research, where there are many open questions. It can also be useful in experimental research when the researcher has specific expectations about the results (as in, for example, the decubitus ulcers investigation discussed earlier) and also when these expectations have been used to define the predicted categories of behaviour.

Before discussing observation techniques, it is necessary to emphasise that there are problems associated with perception. Some of these are:

a. the tendency towards projection: 'you see what you want to see'. The way you have been trained determines your expectations. It is of great importance, therefore, to make these expectations as explicit as possible;

b. connected with this is the tendency to form consistent ideas. This can mean that observation data is, to a greater or lesser extent, distorted to arrive at this consistency (the so called halo-effect);

c. the propensity to develop extensive impressions on the basis of limited information (the first impression phenomenon);

d. observation errors resulting from any stereotypical notions we have of groups of people. On the basis of these, slants or prejudices can appear;

e. the tendency to generalise, to extrapolate other characteristics from the basis of limited data (logical error);

f. the inclination to emphasise similarities or differences in the data, out of proportion to their importance, to show how the data corresponds to expectations.

The following passage illustrates some problems of perception.

How difficult it is to get out of a mental hospital.

It sounds rather eerie. You have been hospitalised while you are quite normal. No one wants to listen, no one believes it, not a single doctor, psychiatrist, nurse. Because you cannot have been hospitalised for nothing...

This nightmare happened to a group of researchers. A team under the leadership of an American psychology professor, Professor Rosenhan intentionally allowed themselves to be hospitalised in mental institutions (Rosenhan, 1973). They wanted to find out how well psychiatrists were able to distinguish the mentally stable from the mentally ill. The team consisted of six men and three women. Among them there were three psychologists, a paediatrician, a painter and a housewife. All were certified as mentally and physically healthy.

These pseudo patients told the psychiatrists of the institutions that they heard 'voices', which said words like 'hollow' and 'empty'. (All told roughly the same story.)

The members of the team gave false names and professions. For the rest they told their true life's history. In nearly all institutions where the pseudo-patients had been hospitalised, they were diagnosed as schizophrenic (one as manically depressive). Once the volunteers had been hospitalised they behaved completely normally again. They then denied that they heard voices, they told the psychiatrists and nurses that they wanted to be discharged from hospital as soon as possible. It was very striking that the few people who noticed that the volunteers were normal were real patients..., who suspected that the volunteers were either journalists or the professional staff who controlled the institutions. The others supposed that anyone who ended up in an institution must, obviously, be mentally ill. The researchers learned a clear lesson from the patients: don't ever tell your doctor that you are well. He will not believe you. You should tell him that you still feel ill, but that you feel much better. The doctor will then say that you are making progress. The researchers also learned that you have to be ill, before you can be discharged. The volunteers had to stay a maximum of 52 days in the institution where they had been hospitalised, despite their normal behaviour...

Most of them were finally discharged with the diagnosis 'temporarily lifted schizophrenia'. Rosenhan was not unsympathetic toward the psychiatrist and nurses. But he did indicate that he preferred other forms of therapy to institutionalisation.

A researcher must be aware of these subjective elements in observation. Once they are known about, 'corrections' can be built in to increase the objectivity of the study. Several strategies have been designed to help make the observation process more objective:

a. define concretely and precisely that which needs to be observed;

b. divide perception and interpretation into two separate stages. Observations, once recorded, can be interpreted afterwards;

c. use an observation scheme, that is, a system of categories where one can record results;

d. work with several observers recording the same behaviour and assess the level of inter-rater reliability;

e. use audiovisual recording equipment and special techniques such as codes to find the parts of and patterns within behaviour.

STUDY ACTIVITY 2
Design a list for recording observed interactions between teachers and students during lessons in class.

Apart from understanding the subjectivity of their own observation, researchers should also be aware of the effects that the method of observation has on the subject. When the subject is aware of being observed, the situation changes, often changing the behaviour as well. This is known as the Hawthorne-effect, named after research into workers' motivation in the 1920s (see Homans, 1958). An increase in productivity was seen during research into labour conditions. This increase seemed to be independent of changes in the conditions but dependent upon the presence of the researchers. A comparable effect might be expected, for instance, if you investigated whether the nurse washes her/his hands after every contact with a patient.
Possible explanations for the occurrence of behavioural changes among subjects include:

– the subject wants to appear as advantageously as possible and to make an energetic and co-operative impression;

– the subject forms ideas about the objectives of the research, and tries to act in accordance with them;

– the subject begins to be actively obstructive, through resentment of being used as an object of research.

To overcome these possible behavioural changes, researchers may use 'secret' observation, by means of a one way screen for example, or they may carry out participatory observation while pretending to do something else. This naturally raises ethical questions.

Two designs commonly applied in observation are:

– *time sampling*, where it is taken for granted that behaviour does not greatly change across time. Data are collected by making observations at fixed time intervals or be making a fixed number of observations at random time intervals, the intervals chosen to suit the behaviour to be observed. This allows the researcher sufficient opportunity to observe the behaviour involved;

– *event sampling*, used for specific events which occur less often. If behaviour in a particular situation is to be observed, then the researcher will have to wait for suitable situations to arise. Consider for example research into the reaction of parents to bad news about their child.
As will be seen from the above, the standard procedure before carrying out observations is:

1. establish that observation is the most suitable method of data collection;

2. define the kind of behaviour which is to be observed;

3. indicate which kind of contact between observer and observed is most desirable;

4. develop a reliable, structured observation guide;

5. choosing a design, either event or time sampling;

6. carrying out a pilot-study to check whether the method works as expected.

7.3.2 Questions

What seems simpler than just asking a question? A question is posed, an answer is given and the researchers find out exactly what they wanted to know. However, it is not that simple. Consider for example:

– the willingness of a respondent to answer socially sensitive questions like 'are you stingy?' or 'are you ever incontinent?'

– the honesty of the respondent, and the care taken in making an answer. The relationship between the questioner and the respondent is important here. If the respondent is in any way dependent on the questioner then this will affect their answer. Think for example of the differences which might occur in patients' answers to questions about quality of care depending on whether they are asked during their stay in hospital or following discharge;

– the possibility that the researcher will direct the subject towards certain answers;

– the perception of the respondent in assessing the questioner. Is there foreknowledge of the aim of the research, and of the answers that are desirable. This phenomenon might occur, for instance, during a medical examination for a new job.

Once again it can be seen that scientific pursuit is a very human activity. Material ought to be interpreted extremely accurately, with as little personal input from the researcher as possible. Moreover, there cannot be too much attention accorded to the construction of questionnaires. In dealing with questionnaire design, it is necessary to look in detail at certain aspects of the procedure.

1. *The form of an answer.* There are two possible types of question. With open questions, the respondent is free to respond at length in his/her own words (provided enough time is available). With the closed question form there are pre-determined answering options, from which the respondent must choose. Pre-programmed answering options are useful when the researcher wishes to restrict questions to specific areas and when the number of potential answers is not very great. The method has the great benefit of making the processing and analysis of the answers relatively simple. It is also normally the least expensive form of data collection. The respondent's willingness to co-operate with closed questioning forms is also often greater than with open questions since no great verbal skill is required in giving full answers.

2. *The interaction between respondent and researcher.* Here too there are two possible options: personal or non-personal contact. With personal contact (or the interview), there is face-to-face interaction. Questions are posed and answered orally. The possibility of elucidation, repetition and continued questioning is an

advantage. Non-personal contact usually takes place with the respondent reading the instructions and the questionnaire, and then answering the question in writing. The benefits of this method over the previous one are the smaller time
investment, the possibility of standardisation and the opportunity to reach
larger groups. An important drawback, however, can be the lack of response.
Sometimes a hybrid of both methods is used, the researcher explaining the questionnaire to large groups of respondents and answering any questions. Subsequently the respondents fill out the questionnaires. This hybrid method can
achieve a high response.

3. *The context in which questions are asked.* This sometimes plays a decisive part in
determining the answers which will be given to questions. The researcher should
carefully consider the way respondents might see this context. Factors which might
affect responses include:
    – what does the respondent think are the motives of the researcher in asking
certain questions?
    – how does the respondent believe that the data will be used?
    – is there an emotional charge attached to the questions asked, either in the form
or the content?
In general, the researcher must try to make the respondents understand that the
investigation is unprejudiced and objective, and that an important social objective is
being pursued.

4. *The characteristics of a good question.* It is, of course, a key requirement that
questions should be well formulated. Factors include unambiguousness, concise-
ness of formulation, lucidity, comprehensibility, and absence of ambiguity.

7.3.3 Measurement
It could be said quite justifiably, that 'observation' and 'questioning' are methods of
measurement. However, in this section, measurement means specifically 'the
attribution of figures to human beings and human behaviour according to certain
logical and accepted rules'. A major advantage of giving numerical values to human
behaviour is the opportunity for statistical investigations.
Measuring offers a large variety of techniques. The following are the ones usually
used within the social sciences.

1. *Test techniques.* This is a method by which people can be compared with one
another in an objective and systematic way. Respondents are placed on a certain level
within a scale as a result of their response to the test situation. It must be remembered
that tests are comparative and not absolute measuring instruments. A good test
should also contain a guide to the interpretation of results. Test results can be used
in helping to make a diagnosis.

The following areas can be identified:
    – selection of people;
    – classification of people (e.g. in regard to personal characteristics, aptitudes,
      skills or mental capacity);

- evaluation (test);
- verification of hypotheses.

Study Activity 3 gives an example of a test question which might be used to test mental capacity for solving complex problems.

STUDY ACTIVITY 3

Figure 7.1 shows a railway track with numbered carriages and a platform (P). Position the carriages along the platform in the order 2-4-3-5-0-6-8-9-1-7, using the smallest number of operations (shunting and stopping) possible. Distance does not matter, but the carriages cannot pass each other anywhere on the single track.

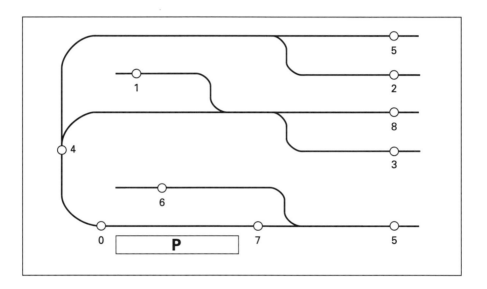

Figure 7.1

2. *Projection techniques*. The reliability and validity of these is controversial. Their underlying principle is that when people are offered a multi-interpretational stimulus, the way in which they react is characteristic and significant. The assumption is that they 'project' themselves in their answers or reactions. There is no correct answer. The interpretation of the results acquired is rather arbitrary. The familiar Rohrschach ink blot test is an example of this technique which is widely used. Graphological tests are also classified within this category.

3. *Inventory techniques*. These techniques are based upon a large number of questions which are used to measure one or several characteristics of a person, group or institution. Examples include tests which measure the career preference of a pupil, or character traits in personality, or psychometric tests, or an institution's willingness to change.

4. *Sociometric techniques.* These techniques try to quantify the relationships between people, especially those which are an expression of preference or rejection in a decision-making situation. The technique tries to demonstrate the pattern of relationships. Two important points must be noted: the result has a highly transient character, and supplementation of the results, for example by direct observation, is desirable. However, the method is particularly useful in two situations:
  – when used to improve supervision techniques in practical situations
  – when used in research to help predict behaviour in certain situations.

Moreno (1951) devised a method to indicate the relationships between people by means of a sociogram. This is a 'social map' on which the relationships or interactions between subjects are shown by links or arrows, as illustrated in the sociogram of six subjects at Figure 7.2 below. This method is very well known as a means of measuring interactions — as are sociometric questionnaires, sociometric perceptions, and sociometric scale tests.

STUDY ACTIVITY 4
Draw a sociogram to illustrate the positions and normal interactions of some of the students in your group using the example in Figure 7.2 as a model.

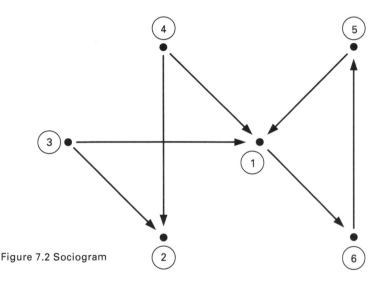

Figure 7.2 Sociogram

5. *Scale techniques.* These techniques require that characteristics or statements be placed somewhere along a continuum by the respondent. They include:
  – evaluation scales, measuring a single quality in a simple way, for example, scoring degree of companionship on a 7-point scale;
  – comparative scales, measuring two or more qualities by comparison, for example by means of ranking in order or pair comparison;
  – attitude scales, where the attitude of a respondent to a certain matter or person is judged. Various scales for use here have been devised by Likert, Osgood, Thurstone and Guttman. For example, when a Likert scale is used, the subject

indicates on a five point scale to what degree he agrees with a number of statements. Thus on a 20 item questionnaire which measures attitudes toward war, an out-and-out warmonger would probably score around 100.

6. *Psycho-physiological measurements.* Psycho-physiology deals especially with behaviour. It studies the relationship between the psychological, cognitive, or verbal aspects and the physiological aspects of behaviour. Physiological measurement is done here by means of electrodes attached to the skin or by other measures such as recording temperature or blood pressure or chemical analysis of body fluids. Examples of the variables that can be measured in this way are heartbeat, skin resistance in the palm, blood circulation, breathing, body temperature and electrical potentials in the brain. The measuring of electrical activity in the brain can provide us with information about the function of sleep and, for instance, what effect medicines have on sleep. Research into fear uses information about perspiration, muscular tension, breathing and blood pressure. The notorious lie detector uses psycho-physiological reactions. Much research is now going into the effects of training the mind and using bio-feedback to alter the level of physiological activity.

7.4 SAMPLING

The researcher must define the group of empirical units amongst which data are to be sought. Often these units will be people. However, samples can also be taken of material objects, for example nursing reports. In other scientific fields samples can also be taken from animal species. We can describe the units studied as observation units or population elements. *Observation units* may differ from the *analysis or research units*, which are those about which final statements will be made.

The group of units which is investigated by the researcher is called the '*sample*'. This does not necessarily include all units which are within the scope of the research. This group is frequently far bigger and is referred to as the '*target population*'. The population then is the group from the target population with which the researcher will work and from which generalisations will be made about the larger group. One possible problem of sampling is in the definition of the population. When attention is focused on all the patients in a hospital ward at a given point in time the definition is clear. But if a sample is to be taken from the population of the single, elderly, with psycho-geriatric problems, difficulties may be encountered. For example, what does single elderly mean? Does single mean living alone? Is living in a granny flat living alone? At what age can a person be regarded as elderly?

STUDY ACTIVITY 5

Indicate what the target population and sample consist of in the Hendriksen research (see the extract below).

In 1982 the population of Denmark comprised 5.1 million inhabitants, of whom 765 000 (15%) were aged 65 or more. In the next century a considerable increase in the absolute and relative number of elderly people (especially the oldest) is expected. Twenty six per cent of all patients admitted to Danish hospitals in 1982 were aged 65 or more and they used 47% of all bed days.

Seven per cent of the elderly were living in nursing homes.

Danish medical and social services for the elderly are both almost totally financed by public taxes. The primary aim of these services has been to help elderly people to stay in their own homes as long as they themselves want to and to 'add life to their years – not only years to their life.' Most of these services have, however, been introduced without primary investigations of their possible effect on the current and future condition of the people who receive them. Furthermore, most of the services have been directed at people with manifest social and medical problems.

Screening studies from general practice have shown unrecognised and unreported morbidity among the elderly. In addition, elderly people are often admitted to acute medical wards because of unfulfilled social needs. Thus medically and socially preventive intervention should result in an improvement in the quality of life of the elderly and might even reduce demand for admission to hospitals or nursing homes.

The aim of the present prospective, controlled study was to evaluate the effect of preventive community measures for elderly people, gauged by mortality, number of admissions to hospitals and nursing homes, and number of contacts to general practitioners.

Subjects and methods

Roedovre municipality is a suburb of Copenhagen. It had 38 020 inhabitants in January 1980 and 37 673 in January 1981. The distribution by sex and marital state of people aged 75 or more did not differ from the rest of the country. When this study began on 1 October 1980, 1376 residents were aged 75 or more and, of them, 174 (13%) were living in nursing homes.

Data for all people in Roedovre aged 75 or more on 1 October 1980 were obtained from a register run by the municipal social welfare authorities. Six hundred elderly people living in their own homes were chosen at random and were further divided at random into two groups, an intervention group and a control group, with 300 subjects in each. Married couples were regarded as two subjects but always belonged to the same group.

The study covered three years, from 1 October 1980 to 30 September 1983.

Intervention group. The subjects in the intervention group were visited in their own homes having received written and verbal information about the purpose and methods of the study. (The study was planned in accordance with the Helsinki Declaration II.) An interview was carried out using a structured questionnaire, and information on social and health conditions was collected. Furthermore, both positive and negative circumstances of the participants' lives were discussed during the conversation to develop personal contact between the elderly person and the interviewer. When the elderly person and the interviewer mutually disclosed a need for social or medical services, or both, the interviewer applied for and coordinated the community services. The assessment did not include clinical examinations. Apart from assessing and advising, the interviewers did not interfere in the provision of services.

Corresponding visits were made every three months throughout the study (maximum 12 visits). Every visit lasted 0.5–1.5 hours. Between the visits the participants could contact the interviewers by telephone to arrange extra visits.

Of the 300 elderly people selected to be in the intervention group 13 (4%) did not want to participate in the first interview and two were omitted. Table I shows the age, sex, and marital state of the remaining 285 subjects in the intervention group.

The elderly people in the control group were not informed or contacted until three months before the end of the study, during which they had received the usual social and medical support from the community.

At the time of the last interviews in the intervention group the controls were visited at home. After they had given their informed consent they were interviewed using a questionnaire corresponding to the one used in the intervention group.

Two hundred and six controls were still living in their own homes in the municipality. Thirteen of these did not want to participate. All subjects who had moved into nursing homes or died during the three years were included in our findings. Table I shows the age, sex and marital state, on 1 October 1980, of the 287 persons investigated in the control group.

No differences were found in age, sex and marital state between the two groups.

C. Hendriksen, et al., (1984)
'Consequences of assessment and intervention among elderly people:
a three year randomised controlled trial'.
British Medical Journal 289 (1984), pp. 1522-1525

7.5 REPRESENTATIVENESS OF SAMPLES

The researcher will select, either at random or deliberately, units from the population with which to work, and these can be described as a sample of the general population from which it was selected. However, a scientifically-sound sample must be representative. This means that the sample must reflect, in all relevant details, the population about which the researcher wishes to make statements. Defining the population and choosing the sample is not always straightforward, as can be seen from the following illustration.

Example

The number of private nursing homes grew substantially in the UK in the second half of the 1980s. In this initial phase of growth, information about them was not easily accessible. In an exploratory inquiry into the functioning of these care agencies, the researcher encountered problems with population definition and sampling, making it necessary to carry out preliminary research into the composition of the population.

An address file of the agencies was assembled through:
– investigation of national and regional daily papers which appeared between 1.1.90 and 31.1.91;
– contact by telephone or in writing with regional and district health authorities and their nursing homes inspectorates

Sampling is necessarily imprecise. It is usually not known exactly how certain phenomena are spread among the population and hence it is not known with any accuracy how the sampling should be composed. This is one source of potential

errors and inaccuracies in the research. Mistakes can also occur during other phases of the research process. For instance:
- measuring techniques may be unreliable and inconsistent;
- mistakes may occur during processing of data, such as input errors in feeding data into a computer;
- results may be distorted because subjects unintentionally give wrong answers or give answers which they believe the researcher expects.

It is vital that the researcher overcomes these sources of error by taking care in the design of data collection methods and, where this may not be possible, by maintaining awareness of the potential occurrence of distortions.

7.6 SAMPLE SIZE
The size of the sample depends on a number of factors:
- the degree of accuracy which is required; the greater the need for accuracy the greater the sample size. This rule of thumb does not apply in the case of an experimental scheme (see also section 7.8);
- the number of variables that are involved in the research and the number of possible responses per variable; the more variables there are involved in the research, the larger the sample should be;
- the distribution of the characteristics to be investigated throughout the population; in other words, the heterogeneity of the population. The more heterogeneous the population, the larger a sample must be to give a reliable reflection of all the various characteristics.

It should be stressed that the sample size is not dependent on the size of the population as there is a point at which further sampling will not increase reliability of the findings. The degree of accuracy is not greatly altered whether a sample of 1000 is taken from a population of 60,000 or 6,000,000.

7.7 TYPES OF SAMPLES
Sampling can take place in different ways, depending on how the phenomenon being investigated is distributed throughout the population. Some of the common ways of sampling are as follows.

1. *Random* (non-selective) *sampling*. Each unit of the population has an equal chance of being selected for a random sample. The choice of units is made entirely by chance. There is no principle of selection underlying the choice, and no link between the units chosen and the variables measured. The sample is a fairly accurate reflection of the population, and it offers the great advantage that it is possible to arrive at reliable statements of probability; connections found in the sample correspond with a high degree of probability to connections in the population.
The random sample is suitable for studies where there is a large number of variables and little information about possible connections between them.

2 *Systematic sample.* This is essentially a variant of the random sample. It is made up according to a system established beforehand. For example, choosing every 12th card from a card-index file would give a systematic sample. This is still a non-selective method of composition.

3. *Stratified sample.* A sample can also be stratified by dividing the population into sub-populations (layers or strata) and then including a part of each sub-population. In this way it can be ensured that a particular variable in the population is precisely reflected in the sample. This can be done, for example, with income, number of years of experience of nursing, etc. One reason for using a stratified sample might be limited size of a population. Another reason might be to avoid over-representation of certain layers or groups.

Example
If an inquiry were to be made into the effects of different ways of dealing with incontinence on the comfort of users, the sub-population using absorbent pads would be heavily over-represented, and the sub-population using a condom catheter or permanent catheter heavily under-represented.
In these circumstances it would be better to perform a stratified sample in which, for example, 33% of those questioned used incontinence pads, 33% a permanent catheter and 33% a condom catheter. Within each sub-population the random selection criterion can be maintained.

Less frequently used methods of sampling include:
– the *quota-sample*. Here it is not the respondents themselves who are selected, but the conditions they have to meet. For example, men of 41-50 years old with a history of myocardial infarction, might be sought. Anyone who meets the necessary combination of conditions might be included in the sample;
– the *area sample*. In this situation the geographical area connected with the research is divided into smaller areas. Samples are taken from these small areas and the necessary data collected. When a random sample of the areas is first taken, and random samples of subjects from within the selected areas only are included, the term *cluster sampling* is used. This method is little used, but it can be considered for epidemiological or market orientated-research in certain fields;
– *panel studies*. With this method a regular sample is used for repeated questioning. This is especially important for longitudinal research (which inquires into change over the course of time).

7.8 SAMPLE AND RESEARCH TYPE
Apart from the link between the selection methods used and the variables to be measured, there is another important consideration in choosing a certain method of sampling. This is the research type. In descriptive and exploratory research, non-selective choice will be used far more, as a particular population is to be investigated.

Example
If research is to be conducted into the care problems which are encountered among elderly people living at home, it is necessary to investigate which care problems occur among this population and what their extent is. Thus the option of a sample stratified on the basis of problems of care is ruled out.

When the results of an investigation are presented, a clear indication should be given of the characteristics of the population which has been investigated, because any statements which are made can only be applied to a population which has the same characteristics. In a test-orientated investigation, the situation is different. If the effect of team nursing on the quality of patient care is to be measured, one ward (or a maximum of two) with team nursing and one (or two) without team nursing will be selected. The results of experimental research are by and large more generally valid, and not unique to a certain population.

For such testing it is important that the two groups are identical or comparable, so that any differences that may have been established can be attributed to the characteristic that was deliberately varied. Random selection can thus be used in both groups, but matching of pairs can also be used. This method aims to ensure that particular characteristics are represented equally in both groups. Pairs possessing characteristics to a similar degree are matched up, and then one of the pair is assigned to each group.

STUDY ACTIVITY 6

Analyse the Hendriksen article (the text extract given near the beginning of this chapter) using the information provided in this and the previous chapters about:
- research problem and definition of terms;
- research type, design and strategy;
- measuring techniques;
- sampling.

7.9 RESPONSE

Once a researcher has mapped out the population and defined the sample, the next point to be addressed is the readiness of individuals to co-operate with an investigation. If people are approached personally and asked to participate in an investigation, a greater willingness to participate can be expected than if they are sent a questionnaire with a written explanation. In the latter case a 60% response rate is considered to be acceptable.

It is, finally, the actual group which responds which produces the data. The relationship between the sample group originally selected and the actual sample which responds determines whether this sample is adequate or whether it should be expanded. When an impression has been formed of the proportion of the group which has responded (the *response rate*) it can be judged whether the sample remains representative of the population. This is important in considering whether conclusions can be generalised. Often however it is impossible to make this judgement. This is certainly the case for questionnaires which have been sent out. It is legitimate to ask whether this is a case of a systematic anomaly, if for example a particular group does not respond because the questions are considered too complex in phrasing.

7.10 SUMMARY

This chapter addressed the data collection phase of the research process. There are several techniques for collecting data. Observation, questioning and measuring are the three basic categories. For each of these categories an outline and examples of possible advantages and disadvantages have been given. Measuring refers here to a quantitative approach to phenomena. This also includes intelligence testing.These techniques can be applied to direct data sources as well as indirect ones.

The concepts of the target population and sample, and the meanings of observation unit and analysis or investigation unit were also discussed.

A scientifically-sound sample should be representative. This ought to result from the size of the sample. Sampling can be undertaken in different ways and the various methods of sampling were discussed.

8

RELIABILITY AND VALIDITY

8.1 INTRODUCTION

Reliability and validity are fundamental requirements of good research and are necessary characteristics of a good measuring technique. Both concepts refer to the degree of correspondence between a phenomenon or concept as described in the research, and the actual phenomenon or concept as it occurred in reality.

The greater the reliability and validity of an investigation, the greater the quality of the research, because obstructive and irrelevant phenomena play a less significant role.

Example

Often, as part of a written inquiry, the income of interviewees is asked for, as a means of gauging their social status. There are many reasons to distrust the accuracy or reliability of the replies to these questions.

Some interviewees may look upon the interviewer as a covert representative of the Inland Revenue and decide to state a figure somewhat lower than the actual one. Others, on the other hand, may give a higher figure to impress the interviewer.

8.2 RELIABILITY

Reliability refers to the degree of consistency and repeatability of a data collection instrument. When referring to a measuring instrument or procedure, it means the degree to which the instrument can be depended upon to yield consistent results upon repeated applications. Reliability involves the identification and reduction of the impact of factors which are accidental or superfluous, and the avoidance of approaching results in an irresponsible manner.

In other words, reliability can be defined as the accuracy of the data in terms of stability and precision. A reliable piece of research yields almost identical data when it investigates the same characteristics twice under the same circumstances.

It is possible that different results might occur during repeated research. A clear distinction should be made, however, between a *systematic* mistake and a *chance* error. A systematic error is due to a mistake in the research strategy or the measuring technique. A chance mistake occurs when a change of circumstance leads to a chance anomaly.

The reliability of a technique is indicated by a correlation measure which varies between 0 and 1. For instance, a correlation of 0.9 means that there is an 81% chance that the same scores will be found across two tests (0.9 x 0.9 x 100). The general rule is that correlation figures are acceptable above 0.8 (64% chance of the same result). Correlation measures are returned to again in Chapter 9.

In the social sciences the establishing of reliability is more difficult than in the natural sciences, where a test can be repeated under exactly the same conditions.
A number of problems relating to reliability will be briefly outlined here.

a. Some phenomena may only occur once, for example the rise of Fascism in the 1930s or the 'discovery' of a tribe of natives in the Amazon jungle.

b. Often it is psychologically or ethically impossible to subject people to the same research more than once. Interviewing someone twice, using different interviewers, would not necessarily establish the reliability of the interviewers.

c. People may be changed by the impact of the research, so repetition would not yield reliable data. In the case of experimental research the 'post-test-only' design is used when it is expected that the 'pre-test' would provide the subject with foreknowledge.

d. The phenomenon to be measured changes in the course of time. For example, aggressive behaviour may increase among children as a result of seeing certain films.

Reliability can be seen in terms of the premise that the result should *not* be affected by:

1. the observer. Irrespective of the person who conducts the research, the scores ought to remain the same;

2. the sample that is taken. If a similar sample is used, the same scores should be arrived at;

3. the technique. When a similar technique is used or when a similar kind of research gives the same results, then this is a sign of reliability;

4. the timing of sampling. It should be noted here that where a phenomenon is expected to change over time, this rule does not apply. If it appears that the timing does affect the results, the research question ought to be revised (possibly in the light of relevant reading);

5. the situation in which the research takes place. However, as for the timing of the sample, if there are factors such as weather which obviously change the phenomenon, this rule does not apply;

6. the precision or accuracy of the technique. As an inquiry or technique gathers more relevant information, so chance factors are excluded and reliability increases.

STUDY ACTIVITY 1
The following research descriptions refer to research which may yield unreliable data.

1. Questions about the attitude of subjects towards ethnic minorities, when some of the questioners come from minority ethnic groups themselves.
2. Research into the satisfaction of hospital patients on the day of their discharge.
3. The same research as in 2 above, using a questionnaire issued by the senior nurse of the ward.
4. The measuring of the body weight of a patient who has been anorexic, using bathroom scales which operate by means of a steel spring which can be pushed.
5. Measurement of the depression among psychiatric patients in autumn.

a. From the descriptions, indicate which factors may be responsible for the unreliability.

b. How might reliability be enhanced in each of these examples?

There are certain techniques which can be used to assess the reliability of a technique.

1. *Test-retest method.* If a technique is used repeatedly in comparable conditions the reliability will be seen from comparison of the scores. In the social sciences, as we have seen, it is more difficult than in the physical sciences to conduct a second test in identical conditions.

2. *Parallel form method.* This uses another test, different from the original technique, which measures the phenomenon in a comparable way (equal conceptual validity). Sometimes parallel form reliability is achieved by having two forms of the same test, which have been developed and tested to ensure equivalence. Where observation rather than tests are involved, parallel form reliability is checked by having two observers record the data independently but simultaneously. Their records are then compared. This is usually described as *interrater reliability*.

3. *Split-half method.* This is done by splitting a study into two parts, in such a way that the two halves can be compared. These yield results which can be mutually correlated, giving a measure of reliability.

8.3 VALIDITY

The validity of an inquiry relates to the real value of the results. Validity is a crucially important characteristic of good research. Without it, research is worthless. It can be described as, *the extent to which an inquiry actually measures that which it is designed to measure.*

Obviously, this means that unreliable research cannot be assessed for validity, because it is not known whether that which is being measured is actually a correct, stable and consistent reflection of what it was proposed to measure. However, measurement of a certain phenomenon can consistently yield reliable, stable results, yet the way in which the phenomenon is measured may still not be valid.

To give a well-known example, estimating the weight of people from their shoe size may give reliable scores, but this is certainly not a valid method of measuring weight.

STUDY ACTIVITY 2

Make up a number of examples from which it appears that invalid research can indeed be reliable. Discuss the examples in your tutorial or study group.

The definition of validity can be broken into a number of different aspects. An inquiry derives its entire validity from one or more, usually several, of these aspects.

1. *Content validity.* This is the only one which precedes the actual collection of data. Its central question is 'to what degree does this inquiry or technique measure

or address the concept we want to measure?' This is a question not only of what the technique measures, but also of what it does not measure. Content validity deals with the conversion of the concepts used in the question into concrete forms and research questions. This form of validity cannot be numerically expressed. The argument behind the choices in the construction of the research is crucial. Consultation with experts in the chosen field to guarantee the content validity during the development of a research plan is to be recommended. In more sophisticated approaches the 'operational' concepts being measured are examined to ascertain if they accurately reflect the 'theoretical' concepts or constructs being suggested; this is referred to as *construct validity*.

STUDY ACTIVITY 3
(for a student group to investigate content validity)
Each of the students in the group tries to define as accurately as possible what they mean by a nursing concept (such as, for instance, self-reliance) aiming towards the development of an inquiry into this phenomenon. The various definitions can be compared, and an attempt made to arrive at the best possible definition of the concept through mutual agreement.

2. *Face validity*. The term 'face validity' is similar in meaning to content validity, but here the focus is on a superficial inspection of the technique. Face validity is therefore regarded as weaker than content validity. It is essentially based on an intuitive judgement as to whether the test measures what it claims to measure. This approach should not be underestimated, particularly when the judgement is made by informed individuals; here the term *expert validity* is often used.

3. *Internal validity*. This refers to the quality of conclusions which may be drawn from the particular research design. The researchers will make decisions, in developing their technique, to measure certain things and not to measure others. These depend on the way the question has been structured and what choices have already been made about the manner of data collection (see also Chapter 6). All of these choices are intimately related to the internal validity of the research. It is important to note that internal validity may be assessed from a statistical viewpoint or from a formal/logical viewpoint.

It can be argued that the internal validity gauges the strength of the research design, looking at the extent to which concepts are properly converted and potentially impeding factors are eliminated. On this basis it may be permissible to apply some statistical methods and not to apply others.

4. *External validity*. External validity follows on from internal validity. The question here is of how far the valid conclusions of the research can be generalised beyond the finding for the sample in the study, in terms of:
   - concepts (concept validity);
   - populations (population validity);
   - situations (ecological validity).

It may be said that the degree of external validity determines the extent to which the findings of a particular inquiry can be applied to a general theoretical concept, the whole population, and situations generally.

Example
A technique is developed and used to measure the risk of pressure sores (decubitus ulcers).
To assess the validity of the concept, the degree to which this technique measures pressure sores and distinguishes this skin defect from other skin defects must be established.
To assess the population validity, the extent to which the results acquired can be applied to all comparable patients at risk from pressure sores, both young and elderly, must be established. To assess the ecological validity, questions of the possible application of the results to, for example, different kinds of institutions, among patients in wheelchairs and those confined to bed must be answered.

5. *Criterion validity.* This focuses on practical utility. Two kinds of criterion validity can be distinguished:
– *concurrent validity* refers to the correspondence of test scores to some other criterion. When these data are collected at the same time and the test scores accurately reflect the other criterion, a concurrent (simultaneous) validity is established. (This happens for instance, when a study test closely correlates with the report grades scored by a group of pupils);
– *predictive validity* relates to the ability to predict from the results that have been acquired. This validity can be expressed in a statistical correlation between actual and predicted scores. Areas of application include school and career choice and professional aptitude. Within nursing, areas of application include risk-groups facing certain self-care problems, or the degree of success of a certain procedure.

6. *Congruent or group-validity.* Here correlations are established between similar techniques, for example when a new intelligence test is compared to an older but similar test or a group of such tests.

STUDY ACTIVITY 4
Identify dsome examples of congruent validity, concurrent validity and predictive validity related to inquiries and tests within professional nursing practice.

8.4 SUMMARY
An effective piece of research requires high reliability and substantial validity. Reliability means that similar results can be obtained during repeated measurements, provided no relevant alterations have taken place in the interim. There are three main methods of establishing the reliability of a technique: test-retest, parallel form and split-half. Research is called valid when it has measured what it set out to measure. Various forms of validity were distinguished and discussed, including content validity, face validity, internal and external validity, criterion validity and congruent validity.

9

DATA ANALYSIS

9.1 INTRODUCTION

An important phase of the process of research is that which relates to the procedures of statistical analysis. As suggested earlier, this should have received attention during the development of the problem and the research plan and should not have been left for consideration until the data have been collected. Important matters influencing the type of statistical analysis include:

    1. whether it is intended to present descriptive findings, investigate a correlation or relationship, or report the results of an experiment;

    2. the number of variables;

    3. the nature of the data. The measuring level is of particular significance, as is the distribution from nominal to ratio level (see Section 9.2.1,a). Only in the case of a normally distributed population can 'classical' test techniques be used, although this general rule is not always adhered to in practice (see Section 9.2.1,e);

    4. the number of samples and their composition; whether for example they are dependent upon or independent of one another, or paired or unpaired. The size of the sample is also important.

Statistical methods can roughly be divided into two broad categories or groups:

    1. Descriptive Statistics

This comprises methods by which data can be summarised in a clear and ordered manner, hence the term summary statistics is also used. The data are classified and ordered, often in the form of tables and graphs. Measurements such as percentages, averages and differentiation are employed, and the links and correlations between data are considered. Descriptive statistics are also useful in data reduction, whereby data is classified and represented in a condensed form.

    2. Inferential Statistics

This comprises methods through which it is possible to convert the information that has been obtained from research into generalisations which can be applied to larger groups and populations. They also include methods for testing hypotheses of differences or similarities between groups or scores and the significance of these (i.e. the extent to which differences occur by chance or can be attributed to a particular cause or condition). Hence the term inferential or inductive statistics is used.

This chapter presents a brief overview of common statistical concepts and procedures. Detailed explanations of statistical tests and their calculations are not addressed. For a comprehensive consideration of statistical tests, the student should consult a text on statistics, such as that by Hays (1988).

9.2 DESCRIPTIVE TECHNIQUES

9.2.1 Univariate techniques
These are techniques for working with one single variable.
a. Levels of measurement
Before statistical techniques are applied to the collected data, the measuring level of the data should be identified. The character of the data determines the statistical techniques which may be applied; this is called the measuring level of the variables.

Example
Consider a fictional piece of research where the following results are obtained: 75 patients who suffer from depression and are all resident in a psychiatric hospital are involved in the inquiry. It appears that self-reliance behaviour, measured with a specially developed scale, hardly differs between two groups distinguished on the basis of psychiatric diagnosis. On dividing the groups according to sex and age, it emerges that young women score highest in self-reliance behaviour, followed by middle aged women, young men and finally elderly men and women. The scale pays particular attention to the time that the patient needs for dressing (the scores varied from 10 minutes to 140 minutes) and the time needed to carry out simple domestic shopping.

– *Nominal measuring level.* At this level the scores are given only a name. In the above example there are people who can be distinguished by a number of qualities: sex, psychiatric illness, etc. It is common, therefore, to numerically identify these qualitative characteristics: each quality receives a numerical label. Thus sex may be labelled 1 or 2, but 2 does not equal 2 x 1. In the case of a psychiatric illness, the notion that the disease coded 1 is less serious than that coded 2 is not valid either.

– *Ordinal measuring level.* At this level ordering takes place, placing elements in a sequence. The groups differentiated in the example above are placed in a sequence based on their degree of self-reliance. Without further data this order gives no more information than that young women score higher in self-reliance than middle-aged women, and these again score higher than young men. It is not possible, however, to ascertain the scale of the differences between these groups.

– *Interval measuring level.* The scores on the scale with which self-reliance is measured might be interval scores. Here too an order is introduced, but the differences between the scores is constant. Should person A have a self-reliance score of 4, person B of 5 and person C of 6, then it can be assumed on the interval level that the difference in self-reliance between persons A and B is equal to that between persons B and C.

– *Ratio measuring level.* In the example, the time spent on dressing gives the highest measuring level in statistics. Only a few measurements in social sciences are made at ratio level. The difference between interval and ratio level is the fact that in the ratio scale there is a clearly identifiable absolute zero and in the interval scale there is not. Care should be taken, however, in identifying zero; someone who is 40 is twice

105

as old as someone of 20, but the earth in the year 2000 is not twice as old as the earth in the year 1000; Year 0 is not here an absolute zero.

N.B. The question of whether a measuring scale works at interval level or at ordinal level is very relevant in the social sciences. For convenience, researchers often assume that the various values have similar intervals, so that the measuring is on interval level. There is, therefore, a wide range of methods at the researcher's disposal for measuring at interval or ratio level, apparently capable of leading to precise statements. Yet a sophisticated statistical method applied to data of ordinal level only produces a specious objectivity and precision. In the assessment of research reports and measuring scales one should be particularly aware of this factor.

b. Frequency distributions

Data can be arranged in the form of a frequency distribution. This is a systematic ordering of the lowest to the highest score linked with the number of times the scores appear. Each score can be listed separately or the results can be grouped. This means that the results are subdivided into classes or collections of scores which are grouped together. The extent of a class is determined by its boundaries. It is vitally important that classes are discrete and do not overlap. For example, when classifying according to age, this may be 0–9, 10–19, 20–29 etc. but should not be 0–10, 10–20, 20–30 etc. The number of classes can be chosen by the researcher, but the more classes used, the more information is required. More classes may also lead to more confused information. As a general rule-of-thumb there should be not less than 5 and not more than 20 groups. For each class a frequency f is calculated. The total of all f's (sigma f) corresponds with the total number of observations: n. It is now fairly easy to establish, by using the percentages for each class (f/n x 100), the relative frequency f' in each case.

Take for example the investigation of the duration of nursing care in a surgical ward shown in Table 9.1. The table shows 14 classes with the minimum duration being 3 days and a maximum of 16 days. Here the extent or boundary of the class is set at intervals of 1 day. (If 2 days had been used as the boundary of the class limit, there would only be 7 classes.) Using the formula f/n x 100, presented above, it can be seen from the table that the relative frequency for the class 'five days duration' is 7/70 x 100 or 10 per cent. That is, 10 per cent of all patients had 5 days nursing care.

The frequency distribution that is arrived at in this way can be graphically presented:
   – in the form of a histogram, structured in accordance with the class boundaries (Figure 9.1);
   – in the form of a frequency polygon, where the columns are joined together by a line (Figures 9.2 and 9.3).

A distribution based upon large numbers of observations can thus be presented with ease (Figure 9.3). The advantage of this form is that it allows for further mathematical development. Several things can be seen from the shape of the frequency polygon; an unbalanced distribution for example, or a distribution with several peaks (Figure 9.4).

106

Number of days	Frequency f	Relative frequency f'
3	2	2.8%
4	3	4.2%
5	7	10%
6	8	11.4%
7	8	11.4%
8	10	14.2%
9	11	15.7%
10	8	11.4%
11	6	8.6%
12	2	2.8%
13	2	2.8%
14	1	1.4%
15	1	1.4%
16	1	1.4%
Total:	(Σ) 70	100%

Table 9.1. Duration of nursing care

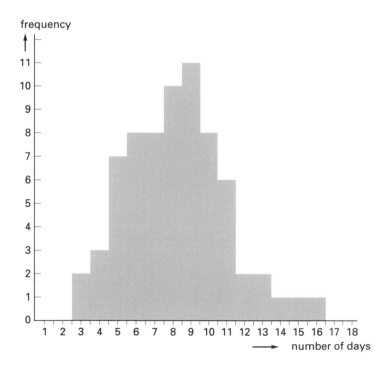

Figure 9.1. Histogram

107

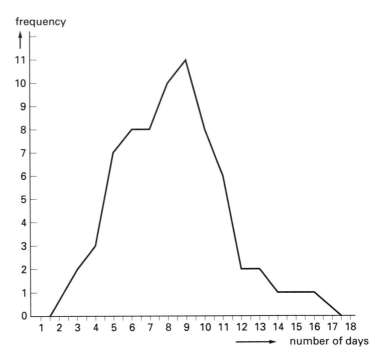

Figure 9.2. Frequency polygon (small number of observations)

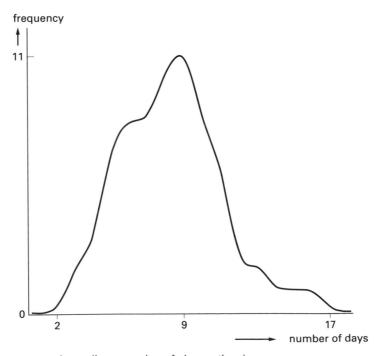

Figure 9.3. Frequency polygon (large number of observations)

A form which often occurs with large numbers of observations is the normal distribution curve (Figure 9.5). Many phenomena (including height, weight, duration of hospitalisation and examination results) have this very common frequency pattern, where scores occur less and less frequently on both sides of the peak. Researchers often assume that the distribution of their results is normal. They then have more techniques of analysis at their disposal. The assumption they employ is; had a larger sample been used, a normal distribution would have emerged. Frequency distribution does give information about one group of data. But if several groups are to be compared, then certain standard characteristics are usually looked for. These include centre measures or measures of central tendency.

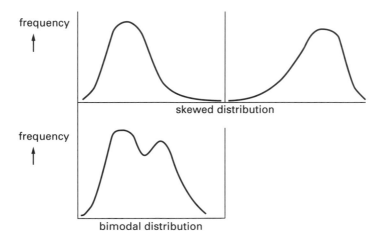

Figure 9.4. Forms of distribution

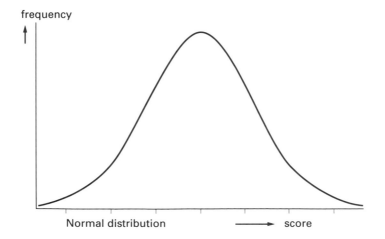

Figure 9.5. Normal distribution

c. Centre measures (or central tendencies)

The central tendency acknowledges that while individual scores may deviate from the centre or norm, the true score is somewhere at or close to the centre. In everyday language we refer to this as 'the average'. The following centre measures may be identified.

– The arithmetic mean or average ($\bar{x}$). This is the sum of all scores divided by the total number of scores. The arithmetic mean is the most commonly used central measure. It will be encountered on numerous occasions later.

– The mode (Mo). This refers to the most commonly occurring value or score in the frequency distribution. For example, the average UK wage would be the level of income which occurs most frequently in the UK. The mode is not calculated by a formula; in a graph of the frequency distribution, it is simply the most frequently occurring value. The mode is little used, largely because of the unstable character of the measure; a fresh sample of the same population often yields a different mode. However, it is the only centre measure that can be used for non-numerical data such as sex, colour of hair or length of training. The mode is also used to characterise a sample by identifying the most common scores for each variable; for example, the 55 year old man, married, with 2 children and an income of £18,000.

– The median (Me). The median is used more frequently than the mode. It is employed especially in frequency distributions where further calculation is difficult, such as very 'skewed' distribution patterns, for instance. The median is the point in the distribution beyond which and below which lie exactly 50% of the scores. It is not very sensitive to more extreme scores; if in the example about duration of nursing care (Table 9.1) one patient was hospitalised for an exceedingly long time, the arithmetic average would be higher, whereas the median would remain unchanged.

The following statements may be made about the coherence of these measures in various kinds of distributions (see Figure 9.6):

– in a symmetrical, single-peak distribution such as a normal distribution, mode, median and arithmetic average coincide;

– in a right-skewed or positive distribution the mode is located to the left of the median and the mean to the right of the median ($\bar{x}$>Me>Mo);

– in a left-skewed or negative distribution the opposite is the case. The mean is to the left of the median and the median to the left of the mode ($\bar{x}$<Me<Mo).

When there are large differences between the mode and the arithmetic average it can be stated that the distribution is skewed.

d. Differentiation measures

Apart from centre measures, which give a summary of the results in the form of one index number, there are also measures which, using an index number, describe the differentiation within a distribution. The following are common differentiation measures.

– Range of distribution. An obvious and simple measure for the differentiation of a distribution is the difference between the highest and lowest score (obtained simply by subtracting the lowest score from the highest). It will be clear, however, that

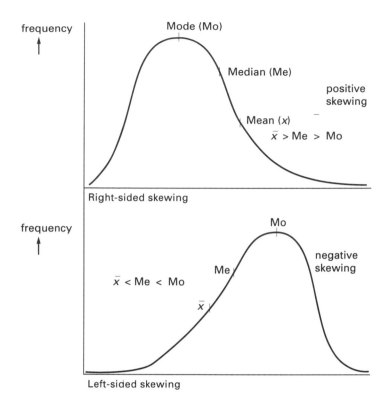

Figure 9.6. Slanted distribution

one single, extreme score can enormously distort the picture this gives.

– Percentiles and quartiles. A percentile is 1% of the total number of scores within a distribution. A distribution consists of 100 successive percentiles (where the scores obtained have been placed in order from lowest to highest). A reference to a certain percentile indicates where in the distribution an individual subject is placed. P23 is that point beneath which are 23% of the scores and beyond which lie 77% of the scores. P50 is the median. One drawback of percentiles is the variation in the differences between them. If the height of the adult UK population was expressed in percentiles, the height difference between P50 and P54 would perhaps be 4cm (covering the range 168-172 cm), whereas the difference between P95 and P99 might be 20 cm (208-228 cm) (see Figure 9.7). Similarly to percentiles, deciles refer to an area with 10% of the scores, quartiles to 25% of the scores.

– Inter quartile distance. The difference between P25 and P75 is also a measure of differentiation of distribution. This inter quartile distance is, like the median, used especially for skewed distributions. Both measures are less sensitive to extreme scores.

– Standard deviation (s.d.). The most common differentiation measure is the standard deviation. This is used alongside the arithmetic mean to describe the most typical characteristics of a distribution. The standard deviation indicates the extent to which the scores deviate from the arithmetic mean, and can be defined as the

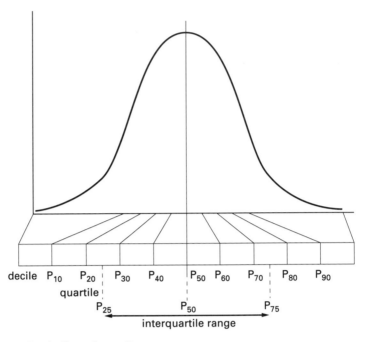

Figure 9.7. Percentile, decile and quartile

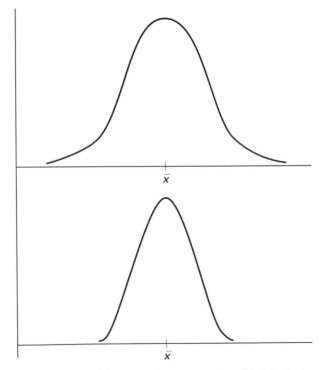

Figure 9.8. Distribution differences with an equal mean, or where x̄ is identical

column	1 score	2 score $-\bar{x}$	3 (score $-\bar{x}^2$)
1.	12	1.5	2.25
2.	7	− 3.5	12.25
3.	14	3.5	12.25
4.	8	− 2.5	6.25
5.	11	0.5	0.25
6.	13	2.5	6.25
7.	9	− 1.5	2.25
8.	10	− 0.5	0.25
			42

$n = 8$ $\bar{x} = 10.5$

$$\text{Sum } 42 \rightarrow \text{variance} = \frac{42}{8} = 5.25$$
$$\text{s.d.} = \sqrt{5.25} = 2.29$$

Table 9.2. Calculation of standard deviation

average deviation from the mean. Two sets of results with the same mean may differ considerably in distribution, but the standard deviation would quantify this difference (Figure 9.8). It is calculated as follows: when the arithmetic mean has been established, the distance of each score from the arithmetic mean can be determined. This difference is squared, and the sum of these squares, divided by the number of scores, is called the variance. The square root of the variance is the standard deviation (an example of such a calculation is given in Table 9.2).

e. Score distribution within a normal distribution

With the assistance of the arithmetic mean and the standard deviation (s.d.) an impression can be gained fairly quickly of the total distribution, and of the position of a certain score within it. For a normal distribution it has been calculated what percentage of the scores fall within certain values.

Thus we can say that:
– within the area $\bar{x} \pm 1$ s.d. lie 68% of the scores;
– within the area $\bar{x} \pm 2$ s.d. lie 95% of the scores;
– within the area $\bar{x} \pm 3$ s.d. lie 99% of the scores.
Graphically this can be depicted as shown in Figure 9.9.

9.2.2 Bivariate techniques
Bivariate descriptive statistical techniques describe the relationship between two variables. Common methods for this are the correlation and regression calculation and the matrix.

a. Matrix or contingency table
In studying two or more variables, the data can be presented in the form of a matrix. This consists of columns and rows where, for each experimental subject, the scores are placed in the relevant position. Each unit shows the frequency of the score. Along the edges of the table the total scores are indicated for each row, and each column

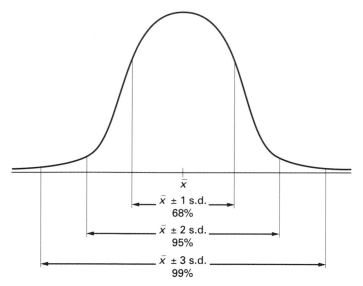

Figure 9.9. Distribution of scores in a normal distribution

respectively, possibly given as percentages. These are called the edge totals. Percentages can also be noted alongside the figures in each unit. This is called the chance distribution of the two indices. In Figure 9.10 a matrix is given to show research results about the relationship between student nurses, types of course (the different types of Project 2000 courses in the UK) and the journals which are read.

On the basis of such a matrix, possible connections can be traced between the two factors. Some tendencies can be seen at once. If, however, one would like to investigate whether the differences are significant rather than random, then a statistical test of significance (see 9.3.2) such as the chi-square test can be used to calculate the possible significance of the results. This is an ideal test where data is at the nominal level as in this example. It is important to remember that the numbers in each cell show the number of students in the particular category and are not internal measures or scores. Tests of significance for nominal data such as the chi-square test, or tests performed on ordinal data, are usually less sophisticated than those carried out on interval data and for this reason are often adjudged to be weaker in terms of assumptions we can make about their results. They are thus temed *non-parametric* as opposed to *parametric* tests (see 9.3.5). The reader is again reminded that for the chi-square test and others referred to in this chapter, details of test calculations are not provided. Texts, such as those by Hayes (1988) or Greene and D'Oliveira (1982) should be consulted for such purposes. The matrix is particularly useful for the presentation of indices which have been measured on a nominal level. Indices which have been measured on interval or ratio levels can also be shown in a matrix, but this is less common.

b. Correlation and regression
There are many ways to indicate the relationship between variables. The decision to use one specific variable is generally determined by the measuring level of the variables. The chi-square test, for example, is suitable for variables on nominal level.

Journals read / Course of training	None	The Professional Nurse	Journal of Psycho-Social Nursing	Journal of Mental Handicap Research	Journal of Paediatrics	Practical Nursing	Other journals	Row total
Adult branch	1	4	0	0	1	1	1	8
	2%	8%	0%	0%	2%	2%	2%	16%
Mental health branch	1	1	3	0	1	0	0	6
	2%	2%	6%	0%	2%	0%	0%	12%
Mental handicap branch	1	2	0	4	0	0	1	8
	2%	4%	0%	8%	0%	0%	2%	16%
Children's branch	2	1	0	0	3	2	1	9
	4%	2%	0%	0%	6%	4%	2%	18%
Common Foundation Programme	4	6	1	2	2	2	2	19
	8%	12%	2%	4%	4%	4%	4%	38%
Column total	9	14	4	6	7	5	5	50
	18%	28%	8%	12%	14%	10%	10%	100%

Figure 9.10. Example matrix

Explanation:
- in the first column and in the first row the variables are entered. In this case, column 1 lists types of training, and row 1 the journals read;
- in each row, scores are given for each training type with the total at the end;
- in each column the data for each journal is entered;
- the last row and column indicate the totals, for types of training and for each journal;
- in this diagram the respondents are shown in numbers as well as in percentages of the total. Depending on the research it may be possible to show row percentages (what percentage of the total number of nurses reads each journal), column percentages (what is the distribution of readers for each magazine) or, as in this case, total percentages.

Correlation and regression are used for variables measured on interval and ratio levels.

Correlation and regression are similar in that they both concern the link between two variables. Furthermore, the same calculation method is followed in both cases. The difference is in the research plan that is being used.

– In the case of a plan where there are non-causal relationships between variables, a correlation calculation is used. This indicates the degree of correlation or contingency between the variables.

– In the case of a plan where one independent and one dependent variable can be distinguished, regression analysis is employed. This technique yields a regression comparison with which the value of the dependent variable can be predicted.

115

1. Correlation

Example

Imagine that there is link between the age of a patient and the duration of hospitalisation in a certain health-care institution: the older the patient, the longer the duration of hospitalisation. This correlation should be seen in the results of research into age and length of stay in hospital. The following results have been gathered:

Age	Duration of hospitalisation in days	Age	Duration of hospitalisation in days
38	6	72	13
54	10	12	14
87	11	56	8
40	13	63	20
73	20	32	4
78	14	73	12
56	9	43	7
68	16	76	17
32	7	46	15
52	7	74	13

When these scores are plotted in a distribution diagram, the picture shown in Figure 9.11 emerges.

In this diagram it can be seen that younger people tend to have a briefer stay in hospital than older people.

From the form and direction of the distribution diagram the direction and the degree of the correlation (r) can be deduced. In this example the long cloud of dots indicates a reasonable correlation. As the cloud shape changes into a line, the correlation increases; when the cloud broadens, the correlation decreases and the relationship is weaker. As the correlation increases, it becomes easier to see an imaginary line in the pattern of dots. The direction of this line indicates the nature of the relationship; if the direction is from below left to above right (a positive direction correlation coefficient), there is a positive correlation (see Figure 9.12). Positive correlations vary between 0 (no correspondence) and 1 (maximum correspondence), and negative correlations vary between 0 and −1.

Squaring this coefficient gives a number which indicates the percentage of the variation which can be attributed to outside factors. In the example above there is an $r = 0.45$ between age and duration of hospitalisation. Therefore, variations in 'age' explain only 20% of the variations in 'hospitalisation duration' (as 0.45 squared, i.e. 0.45 x 0.45 is 0.20 or 20 per cent). If an $r = 0.9$ was found, 81% of the results would be due to the effect of the variable being investigated.

2. Regression

Regression analysis is used to predict the value of one independent variable from another. It aims at finding the line through a dot cloud, which describes the given

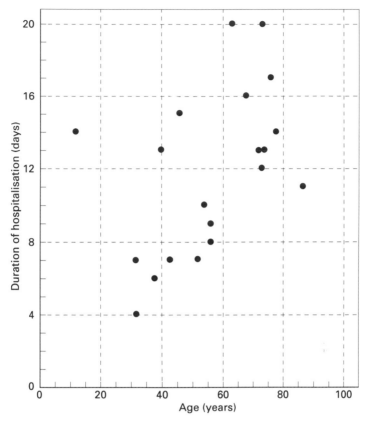

Figure 9.11. Distribution diagram

scores as well as possible. The distance from each separate score to the line is used as the measure here. By changing the gradient or moving the line up or down, it is possible to construct the best-fitting line. The higher the correlation between the variables, the closer the scores are to the regression line. There will always be a margin of error, because the results will not fall exactly on the regression line. Hence any prediction that is derived from a regression analysis should be viewed in the context of the correlation co-efficient (Figure 9.13).

(When the co-ordinates do fall exactly on the regression line, the correlation is 1, or −1 in the case of a negative correlation.)

Other measures of correlation include:
    − association: a measure of the relationship between variables on nominal level (phi; Cramer's phi);
    − Spearman's degree correlation and Kendall's Tau: these can be regularly seen in work with ranking level variables;
    − the co-ordination-biserial correlation; this is a measure of the degree of correspondence between one variable which can have only two states (man-woman; right-wrong) and one factor which is continuously variable.
These are not discussed in this text.

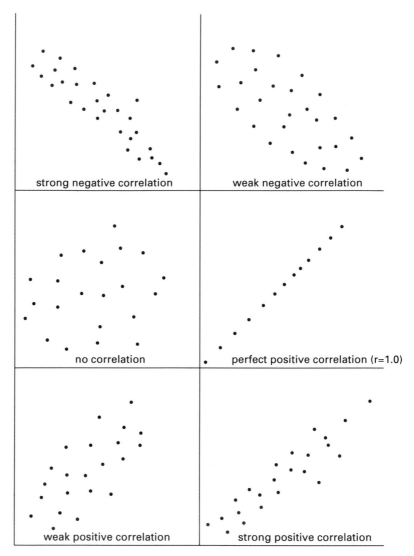

Figure 9.12. Presentation of various correlations

9.2.3 Multivariate techniques

As the name implies, multivariate techniques are used to describe the relationship or correlation between more than two variables. As with the bivariate techniques, the measuring level and the nature of the question determine the choice of technique.

a. If a prediction of the effect of several independent variables on one dependent variable is desired, multiple regression analysis is used. This offers information about the contribution of each variable. In the example relating to 'age' and 'length of stay in hospital' for instance, it appears that other factors also influence the length of stay. These might include the nature of the illness or previous fitness. A multiple regression comparison might then offer a result such as:

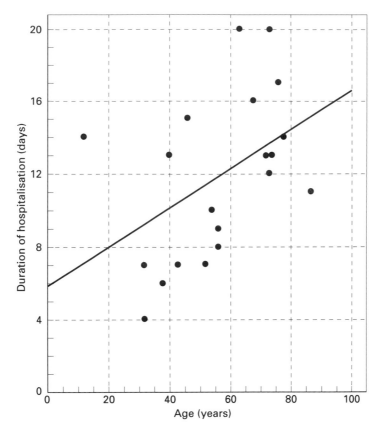

Figure 9.13. Distribution diagram with plotted regression line

$$y = 0.34x + 0.08z + 0.58$$

where y is 'length of stay in hospital', x is 'age', z is 'physical fitness' and 0.58 represents the other factors such as the nature of the illness.

Multivariate techniques also include methods like path-analysis, component analysis and factor analysis. These techniques, which are based on the correlations between variables, are so complex in their application that only the general idea behind them will be explained.

b. If a question of many variables is being used to describe causal relationships (for example in the form of a model), then path-analysis may be used. A path of 'cause-consequence' relationships is established, between the various elements of the problem. Needless to say, this technique can only be used to conceptualise the problem on the basis of serious theoretical analysis .

c. If the variables do not, as far as is known, have causal relationships, then the most important connections between them can be described by means of *principal component analysis*. A form of data reduction also results from this, giving insight into the structure of the problem.

119

d. A comparable technique is factor analysis. This too describes links between variables, but here it is assumed that behind these links there are theoretical qualities. In essence, the variables or items can be found to cluster into *factors*, each of which are independent or different to each other. Thus, it can be found that there are different personality traits eg. introversion – extraversion, neuroticism – stability and psychoticism – normality, which are discrete characteristics (see for example Eysenck and Eysenck, 1969). Using these three 'factors' an individual may be placed somewhere along the three dimensions, so that a three-dimensional 'picture' of his/her personality can be presented. 'Intelligence' is another example of a quality used in psychology which was developed on the basis of factor analysis.

Example
In an inquiry into different nursing situations, various high correlations are found between behaviour of nurses, several aspects of the patient population and the situations within which the nursing takes place. Factor analysis of the correlations shows certain groupings of factors relating to the patient population and the situation. Further theoretical consideration of the results makes it look likely that 'complexity of care' as a conceptual quality or factor explains this grouping.

9.3 INFERENTIAL TECHNIQUES

The analysis techniques which are discussed in this section can be used with various samples and populations. A research investigation seldom covers all elements of a population. It nearly always deals with only a part of it, the sample. The questions which this raises are:

– how can the sample be the purest reflection possible of the population? This issue has been addressed in Chapter 6 and is not discussed further here;

– how can general conclusions be drawn from the results of the sample: the problem of generalisation.

Related to the problem of generalisation is the question of how far the results of two samples can be compared with each other. In other words, how comparable are the samples? Here, test-statistics are used in comparing the results of one sample with those from populations and other samples. The hypothesis, as the predicting statement to be verified, is paramount in this area of statistics. The central problem investigated by testing is: which variations or shifts in the data are explicable on the basis of the accidental or chance behaviour of the shifts or changes, and which anomalies are so significant that the veracity of the null hypothesis should be refuted? Test-statistics can be subdivided into the classical parametric test-theory, and the non-parametric test-theory which does not make the assumption that the observations are normally distributed.

The classical parametric test-theory is based on a normal distribution pattern of results from randomly selected samples, and it can be used with variables on interval or ratio-level. Non-parametric or distribution-free tests do not contain these presuppositions. The tests used here are relatively simple, and can be used to test variables on the nominal and ordinal levels. It is important to study two of the basic concepts which are used here: hypothesis testing and significance.

9.3.1 Hypothesis testing

The concept of hypothesis has been dealt with extensively in Chapter 4 (section 4.3.4). In an investigation which tests a hypothesis, an attempt is made to demonstrate or prove the accuracy of its prediction. In the previous chapters it has been made clear that in socio-scientific research one can only work with probabilities and that absolute statements and truths cannot be expected. A hypothesis may express a very concrete expectation about a phenomenon, but the research will not bear this out. When, however, the difference between the expected result and the actual one gets bigger, the question arises of whether this difference is due to chance factors in the research, or to the sampling or other factors, or whether the hypothesis itself must be false. It is possible to test statistically to what extent deviations from the expected results are accidental, to show when they indicate an inaccurate prediction. However, the researcher must have already indicated, as part of the formulation of the hypothesis, what degree of error will be acceptable and at what point the hypothesis will be dismissed. This is done by establishing a significance level within the hypothesis.

9.3.2 Significance

Significant usually means 'of importance'. In statistics 'significance' is the degree to which an obtained result or value did not occur by chance but can be attributed to a specific cause or influence. It is expressed in terms of probability for which the abbrieviation is p. Thus if we say that the significiance of a test is $p = 0.01$ or $p = 1\%$, we mean that there is a one in a hundred possibility that the result occurred by chance. A common example used to illustrate this concerns the tossing of a coin. It can be assumed that when a coin is flipped there is an equal chance of heads or tails. When a coin is tossed 6 times, it is possible to calculate the chance or probability (indicated by p) of each possible score. (The manner of calculation will not be discussed here.)

Chance of $0 \times$ tails = 1/64 $p = 1.5\%$
Chance of $1 \times$ tails = 6/64 $p = 9.3\%$
Chance of $2 \times$ tails = 15/64 $p = 23.4\%$
Chance of $3 \times$ tails = 20/64 $p = 31.2\%$
Chance of $4 \times$ tails = 15/64 $p = 23.4\%$
Chance of $5 \times$ tails = 6/64 $p = 9.3\%$
Chance of $6 \times$ tails = 1/64 $p = 1.5\%$

On the basis of this distribution it can be stated that if this test is performed with 64 separate coins, a score of 6 tails will occur in the case of one of them, a score of 5 tails will occur in the case of 6 coins, and so on. This might be done to test the perfection of new coins, for use in slot machines for instance. 400 coins are sampled. The significance level is fixed at 0.05 (or 5%), which means that when more than 20 out of 400 coins score tails 6 times, there is a significant, non-accidental deviation concerning the perfection of the coins. The zero or null hypothesis (the coin is perfect) is then dismissed in favour of the alternative hypothesis (the coin is imperfect).

STUDY ACTIVITY 1
What results can be expected in this test of 400 flipped coins? Use a chance-diagram to investigate this.

A significant result always leads to dismissal of H_0 (the null hypothesis) and the area of results in which this happens is called the dismissal area and is determined by the significance level that has been set. In the social sciences, significance levels of up to 5% (p = 0.05) are acceptable. As it becomes possible to make more accurate predictions on the basis of revised theoretical insights, the significance level decreases to figures like 1% (p = 0.01) or even 0.1% (p = 0.001). Probability is often expressed by the symbol < (less than), e.g. p = < 0.01. This is to indicate that the possibility of the result occurring by chance is *less than* one in a hundred or 1% of all cases.

A major difficulty is that of making a faulty judgement when selecting a level of significance. There are in fact two errors that can be made:

Type I Error

Here the level of probability is set too high. If, for example, p = < 0.1 was set rather than p = < 0.05, the researcher might conclude that if p = < 0.1 is achieved on results, then these results are significant, i.e. they are not due to chance. There is, however, a one in ten possibility that the results are in fact due to chance. Concluding that the results are not due to chance, when in fact they are, is the Type I Error.

Type II Error

Here the level of probability is set too low. If, for example, p = < 0.001 was set rather than p = < 0.05, the researcher might conclude that if p = < 0.001 is not achieved, but say p = < 0.05 or p = <0.01 is achieved, then the results are not significant, i.e. any differences are due to chance. Concluding that the results are due to chance when in fact they are not due to chance and are significant, is the Type II Error.

In the technical sciences more accurate statements are usually necessary and only very low significance levels are accepted.

It should be stressed that *significance* should not be confused with *importance*. A difference may be significant, yet be so small that practical importance can hardly be attributed to it.

In the example about the coins the H_0 would be dismissed if 21 coins scored tails 6 times, and also if 45 coins scored tails 6 times. In both cases there is a significant result, yet the differences are obviously of varying importance.

9.3.3 *Classical or parametric tests*

The classical tests are used where there is a non-selective or random sample from a normally distributed population with variables on interval and ratio-level. Of the classical tests the *t*-test and the *F*-test will be discussed briefly.

a. The *t*-test

The *t*-test offers the possibility of comparing averages in two populations where the variance is not known. The purpose is to establish significance in the differences between the mean scores of two groups. It is assumed that the variance in both groups is the same and that the scores are distributed normally. Research questions where this procedure is applied might include:

– on the basis of national workload measurement, it is known that the average time taken to complete morning preparation in a medical ward for a patient who has had a stroke is 45 minutes and for all other patients 48 minutes. Is it possible to say from this that nurses devote less time to taking care of patients with strokes than to others or did chance conditions distort results?

– a group of part-time students attend a course aimed at improving study skills. Before the course, their average score in a test was 5.1 and after the course it was 5.8. Can it be concluded that the course has been successful?
Further elaboration is given in the following example.

Example
A researcher expects that in a certain hospital, on the basis of relevant reading and previous research results, the turnover among nurses on a ward with primary nursing as the form of work organisation will be lower than average. The significance-level for the H_0 – 'the organisation of work based on primary nursing does not affect the turnover among nurses' – is set at 5%.
Research among 50 nurses on wards with a different form of organisation indicates that the average period for which a nurse stays in one job is 7 years. The standard deviation is 1.76 years.
In a sample of 50 nurses on wards with primary nursing the researcher finds an average score of 8.5 years, and a standard deviation of 1.16.
Verification of the results using a statistical programme on a computer resulted in the dismissal of the H_0 (see Figure 9.14).

		Other Organisations	Primary Nursing Organisations	Pooled
Sample Statistics:	Number of Obs.	50	50	100
	Average	7	8.5	7.75
	Variance	3.11224	1.34694	2.22959
	Std. Deviation	1.76416	1.16058	1.49318
	Median	7	8.5	8

Difference between Means = -1.5
Conf. Interval For Diff. in Means: 95   Percent
(Equal Vars.)   Sample 1 - Sample 2 -2.09277   -0.907223   98 D.F.
(Unequal Vars.)   Sample 1 - Sample 2 -2.09393   -0.906069   84.7 D.F.

Ratio of Variance = 2.31061
Conf. Interval for Ratio of Variances: 0   Percent
                     Sample 1 / Sample 2

Hypothesis Test for HO: Diff =)   Computed t statistic = -0.502283
                     vs Alt: NE   Sig. Level = 2.28715E-6
                     at Alpha = *0.05*   *so reject H_0.*

Figure 9.14. Example of a *t*-test

b. The *F*-test
This test form will be discussed further in connection with the variance analysis, and its basic form will be dealt with there.

c. The variance analysis
Variance analysis, also known as ANOVA (ANalysis Of VAriance), seeks to establish whether an independent variable has an effect on a dependent variable. To this end

123

the group average and the connected variance within the test group are compared with those of one or more other groups. If it appears that the groups have individual distributions which do not much overlap, it can be concluded that the independent variable has had an effect on the dependent one. Graphically this difference might be shown as in Figure 9.15.

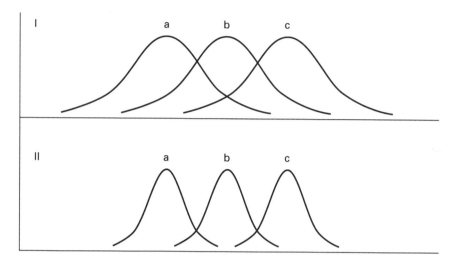

Figure 9.15. Graphical presentation of variance

Explanation of Figure 9.15
It can be seen in I that the scores of the 3 groups a, b and c have a large area of overlap as a result of the wide distribution within the groups. The distribution within the groups is so great in comparison to the distribution between the groups, that it would be difficult to say with certainty whether a particular score belonged to group a, b or c. In II, the variance between the groups in comparison to the variance within the groups is such that nearly all scores can be easily placed in group a, or b, or c.

The variance analysis gives us a measure of the relationship between distribution between the groups and distribution within the groups. If the group averages are very different, results will be significant even if the variance within the groups is high. If the group averages are close to each other, then the variance within the groups must be very small if results are to be judged significant.

Example
A researcher wants to investigate the effect of attending a course in research on the behaviour of nurses during team consultations. The researcher expects that the nurses who have attended the course will report more on the basis of research literature and will more readily 'translate' questions into scientific issues.

124

The researcher distinguishes three groups:
- nurses who did not attend a course;
- nurses who attended a course;
- nurses who attended a course and have performed a small piece of research themselves.

The results are given in Figure 9.16. When the variance analysis figures are established, the variance between and within groups, an F-value and a significance level of 0.0097 ($p < 1\%$) are found.

Confidence level: 97.5

Source of variation	Sum of Squares	d.f.	Mean square	F-ratio	Sig. level
Between groups	3097.1667	20	154.85833	4.848	.0097
Within groups	287.5000	9	31.94444		
Total (corrected)	3384.6667	29			

0 missing values have been excluded.

Sample size	10	10	10
Average	20	25	28
Median	19.5	26.5	27
Mode	0	24	24
Variance	174.667	106.889	58.2222
Standard deviation	13.2162	10.3387	7.63035
	attended course	course and research	did not attend course

Figure 9.16. Variance analysis

d. Multifactor ANOVA
The influence of two (or more) independent variables on the dependent variable is traced by means of a double variance analysis.

e. MANOVA
The multivariate variance analysis (MANOVA) deals with more than one dependent variable (not independent variables as is often thought). The extent to which the dependent variables influence each other and are influenced individually by the independent variables, is demonstrated by this technique.

9.3.4 Non-parametric tests
Non-parametric tests do not start from presuppositions about the distribution of results. They offer the possibility of testing variables on the nominal and ordinal levels. Because the tests can be applied with relative ease, they are also used to obtain a first impression of significance before parametric tests are applied. The following deserve brief mention:

a. The Mann-Whitney-U-Test
This test procedure can be used in almost the same situation as the t-test, i.e. those instances where the difference between two averages is to be investigated. However,

the Mann-Whitney test is not based upon a normal distribution of the scores, nor upon an equal variance in both distributions.

b. The Kruskal-Wallis-test

This is used to compare several group averages simultaneously. This test is comparable to variance analysis within the parametric tests.

c. Wilcoxon's Insignia-test

This technique is comparable with the t-test.

9.4 COMPUTERS AND STATISTICS

The development of the computer has contributed greatly to the fast and low-cost analysis of research data. The computer is capable of carrying out complicated calculations very rapidly and extremely accurately and of processing large data-bases. Apart from their speed, precision and capacity, computers have another important characteristic: they do exactly what they are instructed. This is an important asset, but also a weakness. However, it is not fair to blame the computer. When processes can be carried out relatively easily, there is a tendency not to sufficiently define beforehand which analysis techniques are going to be applied. Instead, options are considered afterwards, or analysis techniques are applied which are beyond the competence of the research question.

9.5 SUMMARY

In this chapter attention has been paid to statistical data-analysis. The statistical methods were sub-divided into two groups, the descriptive techniques and the inferential techniques. The descriptive techniques were considered, and frequency-distributions, centre and distribution measures and correlation techniques were discussed. The inferential techniques were dealt with only briefly in this chapter. The function of the various techniques was mentioned, but calculation methods were not described.

10

INTERPRETATION AND PRESENTATION OF RESULTS

10.1 INTRODUCTION

Interpreting research results is not easy. Methodological and statistical insight and a proper grounding in the theoretical development of the relevant field are skills which are needed but creative and logical skills also play a part. The importance of good interpretation cannot be overstated. Often unexpected situations influence the research process. These must be noted by the researcher, and their impact on the results must be interpreted. The keeping of a journal during research and the use of it during interpretation is highly recommended.

There are no fixed rules to be followed for this last but very important phase of the research. There are however a number of important aspects and considerations of the interpretative phase which will be discussed.

The research is brought to a definitive conclusion by the writing up of the research report. This describes the research process and the results and conclusions of the research are presented in it. By giving a clear and concise presentation of the route followed and the results found, the researcher meets the crucial scientific conditions of openness and verifiability (see Chapter 1). One dilemma which may need consideration is achieving the balance between readability and scientific accuracy.

10.2 INTERPRETATION

The fact that there are no fixed rules for the interpretation of research material is a result of the richness and potential of that material. So much data is normally available that various interpretations are possible. These interpretations are not mutually exclusive, and the researcher can and should demonstrate a broad range of skills in this phase of the research process. On the basis of their insight into the whole of the research process, researchers should develop a balanced judgement of the significance of the material found. It is not intended here to discuss possible working methods for the interpretation of material, merely to highlight a number of challenging aspects.

– Interpretation on the basis of the statistical material

Where statistical data analysis does not yield much information to an outsider, it is up to the researcher to demonstrate the meaning of the figures. Results are only interesting in context and in connection with the theoretical considerations surrounding the investigation. A statistical result is not by definition a theoretically interesting or meaningful result or one of possible practical or social importance.

Example

In an inquiry into the satisfaction of nurses with a certain form of organising nursing care, a difference of 0.1 might be found in the average level of satisfaction (e.g. scores of 3.8 and 3.9 on a 5 point scale). Even if this difference is statistically significant, that only means it is not based upon chance. On the basis of this result, presumably not all wards will be advised to change their organisation of care. (In other words, a result may be statistically significant but not necessarily significant in terms of usefulness or practical value.)

– Interpretation on the basis of the research design

The research design used will also influence the interpretation of the results found. It is useful to dwell for a moment on the problem of causality that may occur in a survey. It is difficult, if not impossible in many cases, to draw conclusions about the causality of certain variables.

Example 1

In an investigation into nursing courses in England, a researcher finds a strong link between the attitude of teachers to the field of elderly care and the time devoted to it within the curriculum. A positive attitude towards caring for elderly people was found within courses where much attention is paid to this field. The question is whether this attitude is the cause of the attention devoted to the subject within the colleges, or whether the amount of attention which is devoted to the subject fosters the more positive attitude.

Example 2

In a survey a connection is found between the satisfaction of nurses in an institution which supports people with a learning disability and the degree of behavioural disturbance of the residents. The conclusion cannot simply be drawn that dissatisfaction of the staff is caused by the degree of the residents' disturbances. Nor can the conclusion be justified that behavioural disturbance in the residents is caused by the dissatisfaction of the staff.

Causality between variables can only be established in cases like these when experimental research has been carried out. Causal relationships may at other times be expected on the basis of theoretical considerations, and in some cases causality is evident.

Wherever one does arrive at causal relationships between variables on the basis of the literature study and research design, through experimental research for instance, the problem of determining whether they are necessary or sufficient conditions remains. Without intending to discuss this exhaustively, the following points should be noted. When a variation in A causes a variation in B there is a causal link between the variables. It also appears that variation in A is a necessary condition for the variation in B to occur. But it is still unclear whether the variation in A is in itself sufficient condition for the occurrence of the variation in B. It may be that this causality only occurs in particular circumstances, or in combination with another variable C.

Example
On the basis of theoretical considerations it may be expected that the occurrence of institutionalisation among long-term psychiatric patients is contributed to by the nurses' attitude to these patients. It appears that a particular attitude is a necessary condition for the occurrence of institutionalisation, yet is not in itself sufficient cause. It may be that the patients need to have certain personal characteristics and meet certain other conditions (of age, for example) before institutionali-sation occurs.

– *Interpretation connected with the theoretical context*
In this area, the problem of a third variable is notorious. A statistical link may be found which cannot be explained within the theoretical framework. In this situation it often transpires that there is a third variable which causes the variations in the other two. One well-known third variable is 'time'.

STUDY ACTIVITY 1
Indicate from the following statements why the conclusions stated are not legitimate. Is there any statistical connection at all?

a. A strong statistical correlation is found between the number of fire engines brought into action to fight fires and the size of the fire damage. The conclusion is drawn that the fire damage can be reduced by deploying fewer fire engines.

b. A negative correlation is found between the preparation time students have for a common foundation programme examination and the grade they achieve in the exam. The longer the preparation time, the lower the grade. This relationship might justify the conclusion that students ought not to prepare themselves for the examination, or only prepare themselves as briefly as possible.

c. It is found that there is a strong statistical correlation between the commercial value of drugs confiscated in the UK over the period 1970-1990 and the rise in civil service salaries. This correlation suggests that civil servants benefit to a large extent from the profits of the drug trade.

d. There appears to be a close relationship between the occurrence of fractured neck of the femur and far-sightedness. To avoid fractured neck of the femur it seems sensible to subject people periodically to an ophthalmic examination.

e. It appears that there is a close relationship between the number of traffic victims among young children and the time of day. The number of victims rises around noon and around 4 p.m. The researcher advises parents to keep their children off the street at these hours.

f. A negative correlation is found between districts making demands on hospital beds and the ownership of allotments by the inhabitants of the district. The conclusion is that the costs of health care can be reduced by increasing the availability of allotments.

10.3 THE RESEARCH REPORT

If the planned steps of the research process have been followed and recorded in a journal, then the writing of a research report should not be difficult. All that still needs to be written are the sections on the interpretation of the results and on relating the results to the question, the evaluation.

However, the reality of the research process is that alterations take place, objectives change, questions are adjusted, measuring instruments do not conform to expectations, and so on. Although the original scheme and considerations ought to be described as well as the actual plan and execution, this does not normally happen. Usually the research report is simply a presentation of the research process as it was actually carried out.

It should be stressed that a research report is different from a research article. The article is a shortened account of the research report. This involves an adjustment to the level, style and terminology, to make the account appropriate to the journal in which it is to be published. Most professional journals have guidelines to which an article is expected to conform. Guidelines for the production of a research report, on the other hand, are closely connected with the phases of the research process. The following parts of a research report can be identified.

1. *General information* concerning the research. This includes:
– the title page. The title, possibly in combination with a subtitle, should be an accurate reflection of the research performed. This guarantees the correct entry of the research into subject files in libraries and retrieval systems;
– the summary. A summary gives the reader a first impression of the nature and the results of the research and will therefore help others to use of the research results;
– the table of contents. This also offers a quick outline of the plan of the report.

2. *Introduction*, giving an overview of the topic. In the introduction the research problem is presented and the rationale of the research is described, as are the objectives set by the researcher.
The research outline is described, and there is a brief explanation of the method the researcher used in the investigation.

3. *Literature review* demonstrating a clear and soundly based theoretical underpinning of the study. The importance of a solid literature study cannot be overstated. The researcher should be able to show a clear grasp of the theory and be able to apply that knowledge to the research. It should be plain that the various theoretical viewpoints have been taken into account. However, it is not feasible nor always desirable to reproduce large quantities of literature in the research report.

4. *Methodology*, which raises the following issues:
– making the terms and concepts of the study operational. It should be possible to fully understand the various terms and concepts in the research report and the choices which underlie them. In the case of experimental research, hypotheses should be formulated in the form of zero and alternative hypotheses. All the research

variables and possible background variables should be mentioned and the values which they can assume should be given;

– research design and strategy. These should be accurately reported. The choices which lay behind strategy decisions are particularly important;

– instruments. Instruments which were used for data collections should be explained, as should the considerations which led to the choice; specially-developed devices such as questionnaires or interview schedules should be included in an appendix;

– sampling. The criteria for sampling, the indices of the sample, the numbers approached, the methods of approach, and the response rate should be indicated in the report.

5. *Data collection*. Given the importance of objectivity and reproducibility in research, the researcher must report how the actual data collection has been done and whether any special circumstances might influence the results. The research journal is invaluable here.

6. *Results*:
– statistical analysis of data. The researcher should give an account of the statistical methods that were used. The outcome, especially of descriptive analysis, can be presented in the form of tables and diagrams;

– the presentation of reliability and validity scores is important;

– conclusions based upon data should be given where possible. These would include significant results and the confirmation or rejection of hypotheses.

7. *Discussion*. In this discussion of the results the interpretations are considered. These may relate to the data gathered and include comparisons with other research results. Here also, or in a separate conclusion, there may be recommendations for applying the research or the need for further research may be identified.

8. *References*. The researcher should obviously refer to the literature consulted and used during the study. These references should be made in a standard manner. A reference entry should feature at least the following:

– in the case of a book: name of the author and initials, year of publication, title and subtitle, place of publication, publisher, edition;

– in the case of an article in a journal: name of the author and initials, year, title of the article, name of journal, volume, number of the relevant volume, pages.

10.4 SUMMARY

The concluding phase of a research project is the drawing of conclusions and the writing of the research report. These were discussed in this chapter.

Three common interpretational problems were dealt with:

– the importance of significant correlations;
– the problem of causality relations;
– the problem of the third variable.

The research report should encompass all phases of the research and the essential features of the report were described.

11
EVALUATING RESEARCH

11.1 INTRODUCTION

To evaluate any piece of research one must understand what the purpose of research is. If it is to provide instant solutions to the problems faced by practitioners then most research carried out would not fit in this category. If the purpose of research is to illuminate the area under investigation through rigorous and systematic collection and analysis of data, then one is likely to appreciate the efforts of researchers in their endeavour to contribute to the production of knowledge. A positive approach to the evaluation of research is likely to make the task a learning exercise.

According to Parahoo and Reid (1988):
'Too high an expectation and too critical an outlook will only serve to frustrate the reader. It is more useful to view research not necessarily as providing solutions but generating further questions in the ever-elusive quest for knowledge'

Research reports and articles provide a combination of facts and interpretations. Unlike other literature, the author is bound by academic convention to describe the steps or stages he or she has adopted so that the reader may have a complete overview of what the research consisted of. Therefore it should be possible to follow the stages and understand the actions and thoughts of the researcher in a way which is not often the case with other literature. As we must not believe everything we read, the research evaluator must adopt a questioning attitude throughout and put the onus on the researcher to convince him or her that the findings and interpretations are 'plausible'. It is useful to adopt a sceptical approach, albeit a healthy one, in reading research. Neither the cynic nor the believer would be able to rid themselves of their prejudices and biases enough to appreciate both the strengths and limitations of a piece of research. If one takes the view of Oscar Wilde that 'scepticism is the beginning of faith' then a position between the sceptic and the believer (see Figure 11.1) is probably where the evaluator needs to be if the evaluation is to be a positive experience.

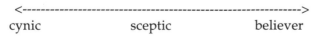

cynic   sceptic   believer

Figure 11.1. Dimensions of belief

However outstanding a single research project is, it has to be replicated many times before its findings can be applied to practice. Besides replication, researchers must also adopt various approaches to the study of the same phenomena, often in different settings before firm conclusions can be drawn. Therefore, while some research may be excellent on its own, one must be cautious in applying the findings to practice before the research and professional community have looked at all the evidence and offered guidelines to practitioners. For example when the Committee on Medical

Aspects of Food Policy (COMA 1984) provided guidelines to the United Kingdom population on dietary intakes, its report was compiled after the findings on diet and heart disease of various studies in a number of countries were evaluated by experts in the field.

11.2 ACCOUNTABILITY

It is incumbent on practitioners to use the most up-to-date and relevant knowledge in caring for people. It is no longer acceptable to base practice on tradition and custom. Brotherston (1960) explains that 'traditional customs are comfortable and necessary things, but they can be dangerous limitations to the search for knowledge and improvements of applying existing knowledge'. The health professional is morally and legally responsible to give the best care possible. Clark (1987) points out that in 'an era of individual accountability, it becomes increasingly important to have access to reliable research based knowledge on which decisions can be based'.

For any profession to develop it is important that it can justify its practices according to a sound knowledge base. It is the task of researchers and others to produce this knowledge and for practitioners to apply it to their practice. In order to do so researchers must be responsible to carry out research with utmost rigour and for practitioners to avail themselves of the findings. This division of labour is, however, more apparent than real. Researchers and practitioners depend on each other.

The Briggs Report (1972) stipulates that nursing should be a research-based profession, and that research-mindedness should be one of the characteristics of nurses. The ability to seek out, read research critically and to apply the findings appropriately would meet the criteria of research mindedness.

11.3 CRITIQUING SKILLS

It is often argued that one needs to carry out research in order to be able to read research critically. No one suggests that a film critic should be a director or a literary critic a writer. The experience of carrying out research no doubt gives one more insight into research. However, it is possible to evaluate research without having previously done any research although the skills and knowledge required for this task can only be developed through training and practice. This book would, hopefully, have provided you with an understanding of research. In order to develop research evaluation skills you will need to apply this knowledge when you read research reports and articles. The next sections are designed to guide you through the stages of the research process and highlight the areas which you should consider when evaluating research. The more questioning the stance you adopt the more developed will your evaluation skills be. Therefore you must give yourself plenty of opportunity to develop this skill, through frequent and careful reading of research.

11.4 REASONS FOR EVALUATING RESEARCH

Apart from the need to implement findings in one's practice there are other reasons why research is evaluated. According to Parahoo and Reid (1988) there are four main

(sometimes overlapping) reasons why research is evaluated:
- For academic and/or professional interest: critical reading of material in this case would be for up-dating purposes. A systematic evaluation of all the main aspects of the study, would not necessarily be carried out.
- To learn more about research: in this case material will be read mainly by those who want to acquire an understanding or improve their skills in different aspects of research. Here, a systematic evaluation would be more helpful.
- To produce a review of the study: if it is part of a literature review for a research project, systematic evaluation is often necessary. In other circumstances, however, a more cursory evaluation would be adequate.
- With a view to implementing findings in practice: for this, a systematic evaluation is vital since it means bringing about changes which may have far-reaching effects.

Whatever the reasons for evaluating research, the exercise requires skills and knowledge as well as a questioning and positive attitude to research. One does not become an efficient evaluator overnight. The beginner may find the task quite daunting. Often an evaluation carried out by a group of practitioners may provide valuable learning opportunities.

11.5 A FRAMEWORK FOR RESEARCH EVALUATION.

Most research textbooks offer a framework or criteria for evaluating research. This consists mainly of a journey through the stages of the research process and pinpointing the areas which affect the reliability and validity of the research. In addition, other issues relating to the political and ethical aspects of the research are also reviewed as they may have influenced the findings. What follows is a step by step guide through the research process in order to draw your attention to certain aspects you should look for when evaluating research. The list is by no means exhaustive. With time and practice you will be able to develop enough expertise to carry out the evaluation without the help of a checklist or criteria. As qualitative research is not necessarily carried out and presented in the format of quantitative research, reference will be made to this as well.

Although different types of research such as the survey, the experiment and the case study may require you to focus more on certain aspects than others, the general principles of evaluation presented here should enable you to carry out this task successfully. It will become clear that whatever criticisms one may have of an article or report, the most important aspect of research remains the rigour with which the data have been collected and analysed.

11.5.1 Title of article or report:

The title should aptly encapsulate in one sentence the main focus of the study. It should not mislead the reader as an inaccurate title merely causes frustration. The lack of a clearly and precisely formulated title does not in any way affect the research itself, but it can confuse the reader.

11.5.2 Literature Review

Research articles limit the scope of literature reviews, while research reports do not. In the case of an article the ability of the author to review briefly the up-to-date and relevant literature is to be appreciated. The existence of similar or related research, the review of their methodologies and findings as well as a discussion of the conceptual framework/s used are all important in setting the context in which the present research was carried out. All these aspects of a literature review instills in the reader the confidence that the researcher has carried out the necessary background reading and is able to make use of what is known in order to further the production of knowledge.

In quantitative research it is customary to review existing literature in an attempt to avoid 'reinventing the wheel' and to build upon the work of others. Where a qualitative methodology is used, often the researcher does not want to be influenced by the existing literature and instead wants to view the phenomena under investigation with a fresh approach. However, the article or report must discuss the research in relation to other literature . The list of references will give a good idea of the use of primary and secondary sources and whether there is reliance on research or opinion articles. A poor literature review does not invalidate the findings but a good one does enhance the status of the research.

11.5.3 Methodology

a. Research statement or question

Perhaps the first aspect of the research which requires serious scrutiny is the research statement or question. This should be clearly and unambiguously stated. It could be in the form of a statement, a question or a hypothesis as shown in the examples below:

Does occupational stress lead to an increased incidence of smoking among a group of staff nurses? (Question)

An investigation into the relationship between occupational stress and smoking among a group of staff nurses.(Statement)

Occupational stress increases the incidence of smoking among a group of staff nurses. (Hypothesis)

Whatever the format used, the author must convey to the reader the precise aspect of the topic, the variables (if any) to be investigated, and the population under study. Sometimes the aims of the research set out clearly what the researcher intended to do. You will be able to decide after reading the article whether these have been achieved.

b. Operational definition

Although the research question or statement may be clear it is nonetheless broadly formulated. For the purpose of quantitative research each term or concept used must be operationally defined. The reader must not only look for these definitions but must decide whether the definitions themselves are adequate. Wilson (1989) offers the following comments

'To take an absurd (but, believe or not, real life) example, researchers interested in what makes happy marriages decided to assess a marriage as happy if the partners called each other 'darling' more than a certain number of times a day. As many married couples know, one can say 'darling!' con amore, or through clenched teeth: as a candidate for a reasonable way of verifying, or explicating the concept 'happily married', this is a non-starter'.

Often the experience or interest of the researcher or the resources available may affect the definition of certain concepts according to how it is operationalised. For example, stress can be operationalised as the physiological changes in blood pressure, pulse rate and the amount of palmar sweating, but it can also be defined as the degrees of comfort or discomfort felt by the respondents. Although the two definitions are different they both must be viewed in relation to how valid they are in yielding the data which the researcher purports to collect.

Qualitative research does not tend to have operational definitions of concepts. Nonetheless, the researchers must be clear about what they set out to investigate, although what they choose to focus on may differ from what was originally intended. However, this is no excuse for lack of clear and lucid exposé of the research process.

c. Sample
Research questions or statements cannot give adequate information of the target population, the sample frame and the method of selection. These aspects of the sample must be clearly described as this will determine whether the findings can be generalised to the wider population or not. The onus is on the researcher to discuss the implications of the sample. The more detailed the description of the sample the more possible it is to decide on its representiveness. This also makes it possible to reflect on the non-response rate, if any.

Although qualitative research may not follow the same sample procedure as quantitative research, the researcher is also under obligation to describe the respondents in sufficient detail.

STUDY ACTIVITY 1
You have read an article about a research project on the smoking behaviour of student nurses on a Diploma in Nursing course (Adult Nursing) in Scotland in which the author states that her findings can be generalised to nursing students in the rest of the United Kingdom. Would she be right? Give reasons to support your view.

d. Research methods
One of the first questions to ask about research methods is whether one would use the same methods as the researcher in order to carry out this research. Where the survey approach is used it is useful to consider if a questionnaire is more suited to the topic under investigation than interviews. The reader must decide whether the most appropriate method of data collection was used and if not what are the reasons and implications.

Where a measuring instrument has been constructed, has its validity and reliability been established?

In the case of a borrowed instrument the researcher must comment on its validity and reliability as well.

The context in which the data were collected is often omitted. The place and time when this happened could have an influence on the data. The reader must also be provided with this information in order to decide how fresh or dated the research is. Any instruments used must, as far as possible, be appended. When this is not done, it severely restricts the evaluation.

e. Pilot study

Pilot studies add rigour to the research. It shows that the researcher was keen to 'perfect' his or her techniques of data collection and was open to suggestions from respondents. This instils confidence in the reader who can be satisfied that the researcher is thorough in his/her approach.

In qualitative research there may not be reasons for pilot studies. However, in some cases preliminary explorations are carried out. Where this is the case, it needs to be described and the lessons learnt, outlined.

11.5.4 Results

The presentation and interpretation of data are areas which need careful evaluation. Sometimes the findings are presented first, before they are interpreted and discussed. This is often more desirable than when data are presented and discussed together, as it allows the reader to scan the findings before being subjected to the researchers' interpretation. Whatever the format used one must disentangle facts from opinions. Not all data can be presented in a report, and less so in an article. In the latter, the researcher will be selective. Reasons must be given as to why the selection is made and what other data were collected. For research reports the crude data in appendices often reveal the biases of researchers in their choice of findings to be presented in the text.

Although the presentation of data may seem a straightforward exercise, the reader can sometimes be confused by statistical jargon or dazzled by the quality of the graphics. It is the responsibility of the author to present the data clearly with the use of appropriate illustrations. Often the use of jargon is believed to enhance the academic status of the article. However, this does not help the reader. There are other reasons why the presentation of research findings may be deliberately obscure. Sometimes there is pressure to placate sponsors. According to Robinson (1991) 'this is a problem with which researchers have to grapple, and the solutions are often to be found in oblique and carefully worded articles'. However, as a result, the reader's task becomes more challenging. It is incumbent on the researcher to present data in forms that are clear to others. The controversy which surrounded the publication of a paper (Bagenal et al, 1990) which looked at survival of patients with breast cancer attending a Cancer Help Centre provoked a number of reactions. One of the many criticisms of the paper was that 'the analysis was complex and the published description so concise that details of the methods' were not always clear (Hayes et al, 1990).

Statistical treatment of data can be used to impress the reader. More important, statistics may sometimes be used as a tool to support particular claims. The way in which politicians use figures to advance competing arguments shows that it is

137

possible to manipulate figures and present a case in a particular light without necessarily resorting to lies. The reader must look at the reasons why certain modes of analysis are preferred by the author/s. Although particular statistical tests are indicated for particular sets and types of figures, often the researcher can choose which kind of analysis to carry out. As a research critic you can ask whether the most appropriate test has been carried out and reported. For example if the author gives the 'mean' age of respondents you can ask yourself if the 'median' or 'mode' would have been more useful. If you are not familiar with statistics you must not take for granted that all the tests and analysis carried out are the most appropriate. When in doubt you must seek the opinion of others.

The interpretation of data is mainly a subjective undertaking. However, a good research article or report should allow you to follow clearly the arguments put forward by the author. There are two 'tests' that you can apply here. First, you can look at the internal validity of the arguments:
Is the author logical in his or her thinking?
Can you follow the steps leading to the conclusions?
Are there any gaps in the development of the arguments?
How consistent are the arguments?
Is the author contradicting himself or herself?

The second 'test' relates to the external validity of the findings and arguments.
Do the arguments make sense according to your experience?.
Does your experience lead you to see different meanings in the data?
Basically, do you agree with the data and /or the interpretation of the author?
If you have reasons to disagree with the findings, you are well advised to read the article again as it is likely that the research may have methodological faults. If you disagree with the interpretation only, you can still 'hang on' to your view and discuss it with colleagues who may help to shed some light on these issues. When reading the conclusions which the author has reached you will have an idea if the main research question has been answered or if the hypothesis has been supported, rejected or nullified. Most researchers would discuss the limitations of their research and would caution against the use of their findings as if they were set in 'tablets of stone'. You should be wary of those who state that they have 'proved' or discovered' something. The realistic researcher would draw tentative conclusions from the data and, with hindsight, would make further recommendations on how and what similar research needs to be carried out.

STUDY ACTIVITY 2
Read three research articles in an area of health care which you have some knowledge of. Find out if you agree with their findings. What reason can you give to support your claims?

11.5.5 Ethics and politics of research
Who funds the research is also important as researchers must maintain their integrity and not be influenced by their sponsors. However, the validity of the research may not itself be affected by the source of funding. What is likely to happen is that

researchers may not pursue avenues which may be harmful to their sponsors. As not all crude data are readily available to the reader, one may never know when this is the case.

Much more important however, is when researchers carry out research to validate their 'hunches' or practices. The personal and professional motives for carrying out research are many. When studies on patient satisfaction are carried out, the patients in most cases represent a captive audience who may feel under obligation to give a favourable view on the care they receive. One can only speculate on the reliability of the data unless the researcher has dealt adequately with this aspect of the study. Sometimes the proponents or supporters of certain forms of therapies are eager to show the benefits of their 'trade'. One can be rightly cautious of psychotherapists or behaviour therapists and others who carry out research which shows that their therapies work. However, it does not mean that their research findings are not to be believed. It means that extra caution may be exerted when such research is evaluated. The test of good research still remains its validity and reliability.

11.6 COMMON ERRORS

There are at least three types of common errors to look out for when reading a research article or report. These are:

11.6.1 Assumptions

Sometimes researchers assume that readers are aware of all the jargons and terminologies used in the text. While these do not always require detailed description often the specific sense in which certain terms are used needs clarification. Some explanations are required for the reader to understand what is involved. For example, it is up to the author to explain how the conceptual framework has influenced the methodology and not leave it up to the reader to make the connection. Often when a research method is used, for example, unstructured interviews, it must not be assumed that these interviews were necessarily unstructured. The author must justify the use of the term. Even when it is stated that a theoretical approach such as phenomenology has been used, the author must give enough details to explain its use and it is up to the reader to decide whether the approach used is what the author states.

It is a common mistake on the part of readers to assume what the author means when the meaning is obscure. It is better to keep an open mind than to assume what the meaning is. The assistance of colleagues, fellow students and lecturers may be useful in clarifying ambiguities.

11.6.2 Omission

By assuming what the reader knows the author may omit certain relevant information about the research process. Researchers are often so engrossed in the research that they assume others understand their research in the same way. There are two main types of omission: deliberate and accidental. Deliberate omission happens when the author chooses what is to be presented. The author may decide that certain information is not relevant and can therefore be omitted. In extreme and rare cases the author may withhold important information in an attempt to support a particular claim. This deceitful practice has obvious ethical implications. More often researchers omit details by accident. For example, if a random sampling procedure is used the method of selection is sometimes not made clear. Describing how the researcher actually 'picks out' the sample will help the reader to decide whether the sample is in fact random. Another common omission occurs when presenting findings. For example, when the author writes that sixty per cent of respondents state that they drink alcohol because of stress, it must be explained that they were asked to choose from a list of reasons provided by the researcher. By not stating the format of the question, i.e. whether it was an open or multiple-choice one it is difficult for the reader to put the responses in context.

You can sometimes check if the author has omitted some findings by referring to the objectives set at the start of the article or report.

11.6.3 Generalisations

One view of the purpose of research is that it generates findings which can be applied to other settings. There is a tendency for researchers to make generalisations from their projects. This last sentence is itself an example of generalisation.

You must try to differentiate between sweeping generalisations and those statements which are supported by evidence. Findings often apply only to the settings in which the research is carried out. They may have some applications for other settings as well but caution must be exercised when doing so. A good researcher will make this clear.

11.7 LEARNING TO EVALUATE RESEARCH

Every professional nurse, midwife and health visitor has a responsibility to learn to evaluate research, even though they are not researchers (Clarke 1991). The implementation of research findings to one's practice is of vital importance if quality of care is to be achieved. Before using findings, however, you must be careful to sift through all the relevant and up-to-date literature. The decision to implement findings must not be taken lightly or by a single individual but by a team who has thoroughly and critically read and evaluated the literature pertaining to the particular change to be brought about.

There are many ways in which you can learn how to critique research. A number of research support groups have been set up. In some cases these groups bring together practitioners, researchers, lecturers and others to share their knowledge and skills about research. These groups take different forms and have different membership. Their general function is to provide collegial support for those who want to know more about research.

Attending research conferences can help you to be aware of the type, quality and range of research undertaken. You can benefit from, and hopefully take part in, the discussions which normally follow the presentation of papers. Many research conferences have cheaper rates for students. Reading the letters section in certain journals and reading the articles referred to will help you to learn about what others think of what is written. You can then make up your own mind about the debate. You can also send your comments as well.

One of the most effective ways to learn to critique research is through a course. Although this is time consuming and often expensive, there are many one-day courses which may be relevant to your needs.

11.8 CONCLUSIONS

Research projects are carried out at different levels and by students and practitioners as well as experienced researchers supported by large funds. When reading research it is useful to 'judge' what is being achieved by what the researchers set out to do. Ultimately the quality of any research is determined by the rigour with which it is carried out.

Critical reading of research is a useful skill for practitioners to develop. According to Parahoo and Reid (1988) it:

'…helps to develop a research imagination. With practice, the individual's sense of enquiry will be heightened as his or her disposition to passive acceptance of the written and spoken word diminishes. Healthy scepticism rather than negative, cynical attitudes will transform a fault finding activity into a learning experience which can only lead to the development of research-mindedness.'

STUDY ACTIVITY 3

Choose three articles from the latest edition of a reputable nursing research journal and assess whether adequate information is provided to enable you to follow the stages of the research process. Is there evidence of assumptions and omissions which affect your understanding of these studies?

11.9 SUMMARY

This chapter has outlined the purpose of evaluating research and has identified criteria by which a research article or report should be judged. Although a proper evaluation will examine all the stages of the research process, the reader must differentiate between aspects which invalidate the findings and those which do not. An inappropriate title or a poor literature review does not affect the data. Adequate and relevant information provided by the author will facilitate the task of the evaluator. The ultimate test of the research is how valid and reliable the data are and this can only be determined by the rigour with which research is carried out.

12

CONCLUSION: RESEARCH AND THE CARING PROFESSIONS

12.1 OVERVIEW

The title of this book, 'Understanding Research' indicates its intention. As indicated in the Introduction to the book, it is not meant to be a manual for intending researchers, nor does it present a detailed account of research issues or research methods. Indeed, in the experience of the authors, texts which attempt to encompass everything the intending researcher needs in one volume fail to achieve their goals in one way or another. They often adhere to one perspective, perhaps covering quantitative approaches but ignoring or inadequately treating qualitative approaches. Often they attempt, in one or two chapters, to provide what amounts to a crash course in statistical analysis, a task which is almost guaranteed to lead to failure.

There are of course some of these large texts which are excellent in parts. While they may, for example, contain excellent sections on sampling, or literature reviewing, or report writing, they may be weak in other areas, such as on data collection, or statistical analysis. Because they are by their very nature large, and by definition expensive, the student is faced with having to purchase more than one such text to ensure something approximating to the comprehensive coverage he or she may require.

The serious intending researcher would be better advised to commence with a less ambitious introductory text which overviews the research process, to proceed from this to more in-depth texts which concentrate on a particular research perspective, and from these to texts which address particular aspects of the research process. When it comes to statistical analysis, texts devoted exclusively to statistics are the best bet and these should be supplemented by workbooks or manuals which provide step-by-step guidance on specific tests or statistical procedures.

Among the types of book discussed above, this text fits in best with that described as the introductory text. The text undoubtedly would be of value to the neophyte researcher who requires an initial overview of the research process. In Chapters 1 and 2 the book addressed the scientific perspective, the theoretical basis of knowledge and the traditional or positivistic scientific paradigm. Chapter 3 addressed the qualitative research perspective, in contrast to the quantitative or positivistic emphasis of Chapter 2. In subsequent chapters the different steps or stages in the research process were described. While these were presented in the sequence which is common to classical quantitative-positivistic research, this linear progression in the book is not intended to convey a bias towards this particular perspective. As indicated in Chapter 3 and in Chapter 5, where literature reviewing was discussed, qualitative research is often by its nature 'circular' rather than linear, with the researcher often doubling back from data analysis to literature review and 'hopping' forward from this to further data collection, and so forth. In the penultimate chapter, Chapter 11, attention was given to reading and evaluating or 'critiquing'research literature.

It is particularly in Chapter 11 that we find the primary purpose of the book coming to light. That is, to provide an overviewing text which will help students and health care professionals to read, understand, appreciate and– where appropriate– participate in the implementation of research findings in practice. This is in fact the nature of this book; it is a 'helping' text. It will not, nor should it claim to, guarantee that the reader will understand all the research reports he or she encounters.

It is a common misconception that in some way understanding research is always a lower order activity than actually doing research. The view is often expressed, sometimes by academics, that those in 'the field'- clinicians, nurses, social workers - should not be attempting to 'do' research. Doing research is within the specialist competence of the academic, it is argued. Those in the field should not be dabbling, but should restrict themselves to understanding, appreciating and applying research findings. This is a gross oversimplification. It is true that doing research effectively is a highly skilled and specialised activity, requiring advanced education and training. Those who are clinicians or practitioners in the field should certainly not be dabbling, in the sense that they would be attempting to undertake work for which they are not competent. However, doing small-scale and limited research is sometimes well within the competence of research-informed practitioners. Conversely, some research reports are so complex that to really understand and appreciate them demands a high level of research knowledge. In some situations - such as in nursing care settings - the need for safety and effectiveness of care is literally a life-and-death issue. The capacity to effectively evaluate a research report and make decisions in regard to applying research findings in such settings requires a high level of expertise and the capacity to make sound judgements.

It is important, as part of the overall understanding of research, that its relevance for the caring professions and nursing in particular can be established. This involves establishing not only its importance but its limitations. It also involves a consideration of how research may contribute to the growth and development of these professions in the future. The following concluding comments address these issues.

12.2 RESEARCH-BASED PRACTICE

Health care in the 1990s is characterised by massive change. New diseases such as Aids are emerging and old diseases such as Tuberculosis are re-emerging as threats to health. Health care technology is advancing at a sometimes alarming rate and, together with social affluence and a more health conscious public, is contributing to lengthening life spans. So much so that by the beginning of the next century the health care needs of older elderly people (i.e. those in the 75 years plus and 85 years plus age ranges) will constitute the highest demand on health care resources. This issue of resources has become an ever-increasing cause for concern, as almost infinite demands are placed on these finite resources. Cost-efficiency is constantly being balanced against maintenance of acceptable standards of care and assurance of quality. Health services are being restructured and slimmed down in an attempt to respond to demand. More rapid turnover, increases in day treatment and shifts to care in the community rather than through extended stays in hospital have become the order of the day. At the same time a more sophisticated public, at least in the context of Western societies, is becoming more demanding and indeed more critical of health care provision. Expectant mothers are demanding choice about where and how they will give birth. A better educated public is more questioning and indeed often critical of the care professionals provide and also demand rights of control over their own bodies. When Ivan Illich (1977) questioned the medicalisation of society in the 1970s many thought his ideas were futuristic, revolutionary and even unrealistic. But in the 1990s the caring professions are under siege, from more critical and cost-conscious governments and a more demanding public.

Professions such as nursing are under scrutiny as never before. They must be able to justify their actions to their clientele and to those who manage the health services. At the same time there is an ongoing intra-professional quest for higher standards of care and excellence. Against this backcloth, there is an ever-increasing recognition of the importance of research in ensuring that practice is founded on a sound knowledge base.

The increasing importance of research, particularly in regard to nursing, can be viewed as emerging from three strands of influence.

Professional influence

This is perhaps the most important influence because it arises from within the profession itself. This reflects an aspiration for excellence, a desire to ensure that practice is safe and effective. In the United Kingdom this could be seen as having come to fruition with the introduction of a new and revolutionary restructuring of nurse education at the end of the 1980s (UKCC, 1986). The new education, entitled Project 2000, aims to educate a single level of nurse practitioner described as the 'knowledgeable doer'. It had been recognised that there was a gap between the theory or knowledge of nursing (itself underdeveloped) and the practice of nursing (largely based on tradition and subjective judgement). The new education would ensure that 'doing' or practice would be based on a sound body of knowledge. It was argued that to be sound, this knowledge would by definition be scientific and research based. Project 2000 would in effect bring together the science and art of nursing in a new integrated whole. Such a notion is well explicated by Bevis (1988) when she describes the praxis of nursing:

'Practice both tests and enhances theory, and theory both tests and enhances practice. Each enlightens the other, provoking insights, altering and changing the form, shape and meaning of each. As the theory evolves, so the practice evolves. In this way, in the truly professional curriculum, each informs the other in the magical whole of praxis.'

Social influence

As indicated above, society increasingly demands high standards of care, and increasingly questions and requires justification for how and why that care is given. This is a significant shift in societal attitudes and one which places in high profile the social contract between nursing and society. Its sharpest edge, particularly in North America but now also in the United Kingdom and other Western countries, is the threat of litigation. This emphasises the legal imposition on nurses to be able to show that what they do is based on sound up-to-date knowledge and expertise. In this regard Hockey (1987) states that:

'Legally, a professional nurse in the UK is held responsible for his or her actions and has to be able to defend them on the basis of the latest knowledge. The latest available knowledge must be based on research because this is the only way by which the body of knowledge can be changed or extended.'

Policy influence

The increasing emphasis on high standards and quality assurance within the health services, in response to societal demands and in the context of the need for more cost efficient use of scarce resources, has also led to an increasing emphasis on research. This emphasis is reflected in Britain by the introduction of a new Research and Development Strategy within the National Health Service (NHS Management Executive, 1991). The approach here is one which stresses the need to link research with the development of services rather than research being an isolated function within medicine or any other professional group. The new research and development strategy is being co-ordinated by a Research and Development Directorate and the emphasis is on multidisciplinary and service-orientated approaches. Within this overall trend strategies for nursing in UK emphasise the need for practice to be research based (see for example DHSS, 1991).

STUDY ACTIVITY 1

Identify a nursing practice in your placement area. Attempt to establish if this practice is in line with recent research findings. You may do this by a library search, by discussing with your peers and/or personal tutor and by seeking information from your clinical supervisor or ward manager. Make a judgement on whether research findings, if they exist, justify the practice you have identified.

12.3 LIMITATIONS OF RESEARCH

It has been suggested (see, for example, Slevin (1992)) that there is an increasing tendency to look to science and research as the only way of knowing in nursing. In this regard, it can be argued that there are many issues of concern to nurses which are simply not best informed by scientific endeavour. Some of these are ethical or moral questions. Others are complex experiential issues, such as the relationship between the nurse and the dying patient, which are perhaps best informed by humanistic rather than scientific forms of inquiry. Such matters cannot be adequately investigated by quantitative-positivistic research approaches. They may, or may not, be addressed to some extent by qualitative approaches, particularly those of a phenomenological perspective (see Chapter 3). Or, perhaps, they are issues about which moral philosophy or theology may be more informative.

It has also been suggested that research in itself has a gender defect. That is, that as science has traditionally been a male-dominated discipline, it imposes masculine forms of thought. This is certainly true within the positivistic scientific paradigm. Quantitative research emphasises objectivity, measurement, neutrality and control. It devalues subjectivity, judgement, involvement and intuition. Even in the debate on the strengths of quantitative versus the qualitative research favoured by some social scientists, terms such as hard (and thus masculine) and soft (and thus feminine) are often applied.

This has particular importance for nursing, within which the majority of practitioners are women. There is a real danger here that, by adhering to value-neutral objective approaches, nurses will increasingly allow their knowledge base to be exclusive of a feminine perspective. Values which are said to be most frequent in women - warmth, love, caring, intuition - and which some would argue are the very strengths at the heart of nursing, would be adjudged as invalid elements of the nursing ethos simply because they cannot be validated from a positivistic (viz masculine) perspective.

To an extent, this trend is being averted by the emergence in nursing of a feminist research perspective. Some nurse researchers (Webb, 1993; Ribbens, 1989; Wilkinson, 1986) are asserting the rights of nurses as women to research feminist issues from an experiences of women perspective. Such approaches have tended to be predominantly in the qualitative research tradition. They also have the strength of not adhering rigidly to assumptions about neutrality and the distancing of the researcher from the researched. However, this trend holds within it its own limitations. Some would argue that in its own way it is as sexist as the male-dominated positivistic perspective. Others would argue that within the new research and development ethos there is no place for an isolationist mentality, whether it be unidisciplinary or gender-specific.

STUDY ACTIVITY 2
Identify nursing issues or problems, one example in each case, which you feel would be best informed by one of the following perspectives:
a. quantitative research;
b. qualitative research;
c. feminist research;
d. non-scientific inquiry.
Provide a brief rationale for allocating your example to a perspective in each case.

Finally, it may be argued by some that research, or science, is seriously limited in the extent to which it advances knowledge in any real sense. The argument here is that

- while research gives the appearance of authentically proving facts, establishing the causal relationships between facts, or proving the 'laws'which govern these relationships - this is all to a large extent illusion. We start out to answer one question only to find that our answer is conditional on the answers to other questions which arise in relation to this answer. As we try to answer these new questions, we find that the answers to each of them is in turn conditional on the answers to yet further new questions which arise, and so on. The task becomes impossible, for we have set ourselves a scientific rigour within our positivistic science tradition which imposes a stringent adherence to sometimes laborious and protracted scientific method. Time and resources start to defeat us. And then, to make matters worse, in the scientific study of human subjects, we are acutely aware that many variables are not controllable. The complexity of human nature is such that the predictability of people is limited and thus the wisdom of generalising our findings from a specific situation is always in question.

This fundamental limitation is well illustrated by Robert Pirsig (1974) when he comments that:
'If the purpose of the scientific method is to select from among a multitude of hypotheses, and if the number of hypotheses grows faster than experimental method can handle, then it is clear that all hypotheses can never be tested. If all hypotheses cannot be tested, then the results of any experiment are inconclusive and the entire scientific method falls short of its goal of establishing proven knowledge.'

A problem here is that we seem to have become entrapped within this particular positivistic perspective. We have come to regard it to be true that knowledge gained through this perspective is the only authentic way of knowing. This has become reified within our culture and we are blind to any questioning of this premise. In the behavioural and social sciences, and particularly in psychology, there is a tendency to adhere with almost blind tenacity to the laboratory, the measurement instrument and the statistic. In this regard, Rogers (1968) stated that:
'In the behavioral sciences, I think that one of our problems is that the methods of testing hypotheses come to be regarded as dogmas. These are, or should be, as unwelcome as dogmas in any other field. Our rules and methods for testing hypotheses are creations of the scientists themselves, and should be recognized as such. Thus, we should realize that there is no special virtue in any one procedure. Some hypotheses can be tested on a single individual. One such famous hypothesis had to do with the circulation of blood, and the testing of it involved no statistics. Others can only be satisfactorily tested on a large population using all of the most elaborate statistical methods.'
Rogers is clearly presenting simple and straightforward common sense here. No-one other than the most narrowminded of positivistic thinkers would seriously refute his viewpoint. Yet in the behavioural and social sciences it is usually only the most elaborate statistical studies which are granted respect and recognition. In the caring professions, themselves aspiring to high professional status and recognition, there is a tendency to hold only this type of research in high regard, because this is what is seen to be important and scientifically respectable.

The reader would be excused for reacting with a certain amount of agitation to this apparent devaluing of the scientific method. Why present a book on understanding research and end it by questioning the very validity of the scientific method? The answer is, of course, that we are not endeavouring to do this. A scientifically sound knowledge base is essential to the modern practice of nursing. But we *must* accept and acknowledge its limitations. This is not a total negating of science and research at all. It is, rather, a recognition of the sound principle of positive scepticism as explicated in Chapter 11. This questioning attitude, this demanding of soundness and proof, and questioning of proof and conclusions, is in fact a core element in the scientific ethos. To not adopt this stance, to not forever question and demand proof, to not recognise the limitations of this 'proof', to not search for new and more appropriate and more effective methods, would be the real negation of the scientific perspective.

12.4 NEW PARADIGMS IN RESEARCH
Towards new approaches

It has been suggested above that as caring professionals we must recognise that there are other non-scientific ways of knowing which are equally important in the development of nursing knowledge and practice. Nevertheless, there are aspects of practice which do appear to merit a research-orientated mode of inquiry. However, again as suggested earlier, the mainstream positivistic or quantitative approach is often limited in the extent to which it can answer some of the questions being asked. This is particularly the case in nursing, an activity which is essentially humanistic, concerned with intimate caring and deeply subjective interpersonal relationships. It is argued that, by virtue of its essentially objective and neutral perspective, the quantitative or positivistic perspective is in fact alien to this area of activity. Indeed, this has already been touched upon above, in the context of arguments for a feminist research perspective. We must thus either look to non-scientific approaches, adopt qualitative approaches if they are appropriate, or develop new scientific paradigms.

The argument suggested here is this. If we want to investigate an issue in which the variables are easily identified, measured and manipulated, quantitative methods are adequate. Indeed, depending on the research questions, they may be the approaches of choice. We can, for example, identify the types of back injury most common among nurses and we can investigate the influence of training in lifting techniques on the incidence of such injury. Similarly, we can conduct time sampling studies to establish the levels of activity among the elderly residents of a nursing home, we can introduce activity programmes and measure the effects of these on the levels of residents' engagement. But in reality it is not this simple. Other variables which we cannot control may corrupt our findings or introduce margins of error which question our results. Establishing the types of back injury is notoriously difficult and there may be malingering or psychosomatic influences at play. However, we have means of grappling with such problems - by controlling for these variables or by estimating the degree of error they bring to our findings.

But what if we are interested not simply in levels of activity among elderly residents, but in the meaningfulness of life in nursing homes or the nature of the nurse-patient relationship and how it may be therapeutically constructed? Here the straightforward quantitative study is of little value to us. Here we are in search of words and meanings, not numbers and statistics. But even if we adopt more qualitative approaches, we find that they do not always enable us to get under the very skin of practice in order to understand its deeper, more complex, more subjective meanings.

The need for a different scientific paradigm is thus particularly important in the context of the caring professions. We *can* answer some of our questions by a classical positivistic approach. However these tend to be the easiest questions. The challenging questions, and those which we sometimes tend to avoid ourselves, because of their difficult and sometimes emotive nature - such as questions concerning the intimate nature of caring, coping with death and dying or emotional aspects of the nurse-patient relationship - require different approaches. The challenge here is illustrated by Schön (1987), when he comments that:

'In the varied topography of professional practice, there is a high, hard ground overlooking a swamp. On the high ground, manageable problems lend themselves to solution through the application of research-based theory and technique. In the swampy lowland, messy confusing problems defy technical solution. The practitioner must choose. Should he remain on the high ground where he can solve relatively unimportant problems according to prevailing standards of rigour or shall he descend to the swamp of important problems and nonrigorous inquiry?'

If our practice does, as indeed it *must*, enter this 'swampy ground' it should be a sound practice based on sound knowledge and research. Our research must thus enter the swampy ground as well, in order to map it out and grasp its essential meaning. As the tools of positivistic science are inadequate for this purpose, new approaches become essential. But an important point to keep in mind here is this. So often the argument rages between the value of the positivistic, quantitative paradigm *as opposed to* the humanistic, qualitative paradigm. This controversy is not only irrelevant in reality but dysfunctional to our quest for knowledge. We must not assume that adopting the new paradigm requires rejecting in its totality the old, despite the connotations of 'new direction'implicit in the term 'paradigm'. Both have their place in our quest, as suggested by Rogers (1985), when he states that:

'The Newtonian, mechanistic, reductionist, linear cause-effect, behaviorist view of science is not thrown out but it is seen as simply one aspect of science, a perfectly good way of investigating some problems, but decidedly inappropriate for others.'

New Paradigm Research

Thus far, the debate has been directed toward needing a new paradigm which has emerged as being more appropriate for the development of some of the more complex and humanistic aspects of our knowledge. But what is this 'new paradigm research' which has emerged? It is unfortunately a coat of many colours, precisely because it is new and is in fact still emerging. To some, new paradigm research is a specific research approach. To others, new paradigms *in* research refers to all new methods and approaches introduced in their discipline. But, in general, it is a new and very different way of doing research, one which rejects the quantitative, positivistic perspective. While it is an approach which in general adopts qualitative methods, it is unique in that it does not acknowledge a separation between researcher and the researched. Even in qualitative research involving participant observation, there is a researcher and there are subjects. In new paradigm research there is a tendency to remove these boundaries. And, finally, it is characterised by an openness which accepts a variety of methods, adhering to the principle that the method is determined by the research question and not by a rigid adherence to some discipline-bound orthodoxy of method.

Some ideas or perspectives which characterise new paradigm approaches are as follows.

New paradigm research as 'indwelling'

Here the researcher developes a deep, subjective, empathic relationship with the subject/s. In essence, this is an attempt to get under the subject's skin, to experience the situation as he experiences it, an approach described as 'indwelling'. According to Polanyi (1958), the knowledge gained from this depth of relationship or 'indwelling' with the subjects leads to new insights into the human condition and human relationships. It can be seen that this perspective is essentially qualitative and similar to the phenomenological research described in Chapter 3. However its closeness of relationship between researcher and subject is more reminiscent of the counselling relationship than of that between the qualitative researcher and his subject.

New paradigm research as collaboration

The term new paradigm research was first made popular by Reason and Rowan (1981) and later refined by Reason (1988). The basis of the perspective was essentially established on the assertion that orthodox research methods are inadequate for a science of persons. The idea is essentially to conduct inquiry by breaking down barriers between the researcher and the researched. All those involved collaborate in the quest for knowledge as both researchers and subjects, as in fact researchers-subjects or co-researchers. It is thus not only research but a form of education, personal development and social action. In essence co-researchers work together to:
- discuss the research problem;
- decide on methods of research or inquiry;
- self-observe;
- reflect on experience;
- decide together on problem resolution;
- take action on the basis of findings.

New paradigm research as method

In line with the above philosophy, Reinharz (1981) speaks of new paradigm methods as a variety of methods in the general rubric of qualitative research methodology. However, in these new methodologies, these are further characterised by recognition of the researcher and his impressions as part of the data. In more traditional positivistic approaches a cardinal rule is that the researcher does not in any way intrude in the field. Indeed, some methodologists have drawn up detailed taxonomies or listings of observer biases which if not avoided, it is claimed, may even invalidate the research project. Even in qualitative research it is often stressed that the subjective or personal viewpoint or interpretations of the researcher should be reserved until data or information analysis is taking place. This inclusion by the researcher of himself as subject is not a dissimilar situation to the co-researcher role of the researcher advocated by Reason (op. cit.).

New paradigm research as action

An essential notion within the original concept of new paradigm research as expounded by Reason and Rowan (1981) was that of taking action on the basis of findings. The new paradigm is thus essentially applied rather than pure research. For some, this 'action'orientation is the innovative feature of the new paradigm(see for example Cohen and Manion, 1989). This is often presented under the title 'Action Research'. While there are some variations in definition, Action Research is usually described as being:

– a small-scale study of the real world;
– situational and interventionist, ie. 'action' orientated and aimed at developing practices, policies, procedures etc. ;
– collaborative, with researchers and subjects working together;
– aimed at organisational development and change.

New paradigm research is increasingly found in situations such as those in which caring professionals work. For example, using diaries or accounts is a long-standing qualitative method. But in new paradigm research, both researcher and subject (the co-researchers) may maintain the diary, and their discussions and joint analysis of content becomes part of the data. Here old rigid roles of researcher separateness and non-involvement are breached, but benefits in terms of increased insights and deep subjective understanding are reaped as a result. As another example, a relatively recent innovation in nursing is that of nursing development units. Here clinicians, educators and researchers work together to identify nursing problems. They agree methods of researching these problems and develop and introduce new and improved methods of practice as a result of these activities. This is in fact 'action research' in action.

STUDY ACTIVITY 3

Make three columns and head them quantitative research, qualitative research and new paradigm research. List in each column the characteristics of the methods. You should endeavour to end up with at least six characteristics in each column. When you have done this, compare and contrast the three perspectives. If possible share and discuss your lists with fellow students or colleagues who have also undertaken this activity. You (and they) may be able to extend your lists as a result of these discussions.

12.5 TOWARDS THE FUTURE

Particularly since the 1980s a significant change can be seen to be taking place in British nursing. As indicated earlier in this concluding chapter a number of professional, societal, legal and policy-initiated influences have created a research orientation in nursing. This is reflected in nursing curricula, particularly since the advent of Project 2000 (UKCC, 1986). It would now be unusual to encounter a nursing

curriculum in the United Kingdom which does not incorporate a research component. We now recognise the need for a sound research base to our practice. We now
acknowledge the need to understand research, to appreciate the relevance of research
and, where appropriate, to apply research findings in practice.

An increasing number of clinicians and nurse managers are graduates. In many areas
the proportion of nurse teachers who are graduates is well above the fifty percent
level and in some instances is approaching one hundred percent. With the introduction of Project 2000 all new practitioners will be educated to Higher Education
Diploma level, equivalent to the first two years of a three-year baccalaureate degree.
The nurse of the future will be more analytic in her approach, and be capable of
applying critical thinking and a questioning attitude to her practice. Already she has
a growing body of knowledge at her disposal, as the amount of academic and
research literature proliferates in the professional journals, and as nursing texts
become increasingly research -based and academic in their orientation. It could be
argued that as a profession we already are to a significant extent at a stage of readiness
to achieve a sound research base for our practice.

However, as stated above, this is a change which is now taking place. We are not yet
at that stage where we could claim that to a significant extent research is guiding
our practice in its totality. It is interesting to note this recent comment, which relates
to midwives but could equally be applied to nurses and health visitors, by Chalmers
(1993):
'Midwives are using pregnant women and babies as guinea pigs in uncontrolled
experimentation in their everyday practice. For example, how many midwives have
recommended that women use 'Epifoam', or 'Rotersept', or hairdryers for drying the
perineum; and what unbiased evidence would they point to as justification for
promoting these forms of care? Can midwives point to evidence showing that
weighing women routinely during pregnancy is more likely to do good than harm?'

This is a rather provocative and challenging statement. Yet it carries an element of
truth in it. More often than not our practice is based on tradition and convention
rather than research. If our practice is not based on research or on an equally
acceptable sound knowledge base, is it the reality - as Chalmers suggests - that we are
using our patients and clients as guinea pigs, but in a mindless way, not even with the
caution of the scientist in his laboratory? If this is so, it clearly is no longer acceptable.
We *must* ensure that our practice is based on a sound body of knowledge. This
requires not only that research is adequately funded and carried out, but also that
there is a commitment within educators, managers and practitioners themselves to
developing a research-based profession.

It is essential that in the future our ways of practice are integrated with our ways
of knowing and the outcomes of this knowledge. The challenge of the future is in
essence twofold. Firstly, we must achieve the goal of a sound knowledge informing
practice, and of that practice in turn informing our knowledge. We must achieve a
situation of praxis where practice is, in its very happening, the enactment of
knowledgeable doing as advocated in Project 2000 (UKCC, 1986). Where, in effect,

practice is sound knowledge in action. Secondly, we must ensure that this knowledge is directly relevant and applicable. The nature of academic disciplines and their forms of knowledge must not be allowed to impose upon us the nature and form of our body of nursing knowledge. Rather, nursing itself must determine the nature of its own knowledge. We must be open to knowledge attained through quantitative research based on the conventional scientific model. But we must not be confined by this orthodoxy. We must also draw upon the qualitative scientific paradigm, upon arts and the humanities, upon philosophy, and upon new branches of knowledge where we feel this is appropriate, because we are developing a science *and* an art of nursing. And, where our needs justify it, we must be prepared to try out, to develop, and to use new scientific paradigms where these best inform aspects of our practice. We must not only have science *in* nursing, we must have a science *of* and *for* nursing.

REFERENCES

Aamodt, A. M. (1986). Discovering the child's view of alopecia: doing ethnography, in Munhall P.L. and Oiler C.J. (eds)(1986) *Nursing Research: A Qualitative Perspective,* Connecticut, Appleton Century Crofts.

Anderson, J.M. (1991). Immigrant women speak of chronic illness: the social construction of the devalued self, *Journal of Advanced Nursing*,16,6, 710–717.

Asch, S.E. (1952). *Social Psychology,* New York, Prentice Hall.

Atkinson, P., Delamont S., and Hammersley, M. (1988). Qualitative research traditions: a British response to Jacob. *Review of Educational Research*, 88, 231–250.

Atkinson, R.L., and Atkinson, C.A. (1975).*Study Guide with Programmed Units and Learning Objectives*, New York, Harcourt Brace Jovanovich Inc.

Bagenal, F.S., Easton, D.F., Harris, E., Chilvers, C.E.D., and Mc Elwain, T.J. (1990). Survival of patients with breast cancer attending Bristol Cancer Help Centre,*The Lancet.* Sept 8, 336, 8715, 606–610.

Baker, C., Wuest, J., and Stern, P.N. (1992). Method slurring: the grounded theory/ phenomenology example, *Journal of Advanced Nursing*, 17, 1355–1360.

Batey, M.V. (1977). Conceptualisation, knowledge and logic guiding empirical research.*Nursing Research*, 26 (5), 324–329.

Berger, P.L., and Luckmann, T. (1967). *The Social Construction of Reality,* Harmondsworth, Penguin.

Best, J.W. (1970). *Research in Education* (2nd edition), Englewood Cliffs, New Jersey, Prentice Hall.

Bevis, E.O. (1988). New directions for a new age in National League for Nursing (Eds), *Curriculum Revolution: Mandate for Change,* New York, National League for Nursing.

Bliss-Holz, J. (1989). Comparison of rectal, axillary and inguinal temperatures in full-term newborn infants, *Nursing Research*, 38/2, 85–87.

Blumer, H. (1969). *Symbolic Interactionism: Perspectives and Method*, Englewood Cliffs, Prentice Hall.

Bogdan, R.C., and Biklen, S.K. (1982). *Qualitative Research in Education*, Boston, Allyn and Bacon Inc.

Bogdan, R., and Taylor, S. (1975). *Introduction to Qualitative Research Methods*, New York, Wiley.

Briggs, A. (Chairman) (1972). Report of the Committee on Nursing, HMSO, London.

Brotherston, J. (1960). *Learning to Investigate Problems*, ICN, Geneva.

Burns, N. and Grove, S.K. (1987). *The Practice of Nursing Research - Conduct, Critique and Utilisation*, Philadelphia, W.B. Saunders.

Callow, L.B., and Piper, B. (1989). Effect of backrest on central renous pressure in pediatric cardiac surgery, *Nursing Research*, 38/6, 336–338.

Ceslowitz, S.B. (1989). Burnout and coping strategies among hospital staff nurses, *Journal of Advanced Nursing*, 14, 553–557.

Chalmers, I. (1993). Effective care in midwifery – research, the professions and the public, *Midwives Chronicle*, 106, 1, 260, 3–13.

Chinn, P.L. (1985). Debunking myths in nursing theory and research, *Image: The Journal of Nursing Scholarship*, XVIII, 2, 45–49.

Clark, E. (1987). Research awareness: its importance in practice, *Professional Nurse*, 2, 11, 371–373.

Clark, E. (1991). *Evaluating Research, in Research Awareness* (Module No. 10), London, Distance Learning Centre, South Bank Polytechnic.

Cohen, L. and Manion, L. (1989). *Research Methods in Education*, London, Routledge.

Committee on Medical Aspects of Food Policy (COMA) (1984).*Report of the Panel on Diet in Relation to Cardiovascular Disease*, DHSS, London.

Cowley, S. (1991). A symbolic awareness context identified through a grounded theory study of health visiting, *Journal of Advanced Nursing*, 16, 6, 648–656.

Department of Health and Social Services (DHSS) (1991).*A Strategy for Nursing, Midwifery and Health Visiting in Northern Ireland*, Belfast, DHSS.

Deutscher, I. (1966). Words and deeds: social science and social policy, *Social Problems*, 13, 233–254.

Dowd, T.T. (1991). Discovering older women's experience of urinary incontinence, *Research in Nursing and Health*, 14, 179–186.

Eysenck, H.J. and Eysenck, S.B.G. (1969). *Personality Structure and Measurement*, San Diego, Knapp.

Field, P. and Morse, J. (1985). *Nursing Research: The Application of Qualitative Approaches*, Rockville, Maryland, Aspen Publishers.

Fontana, A. (1977). *The Last Frontier,* Beverley Hills, Sage Publications.

Gallego, A.P. (1983). *Evaluating the School,* London, Royal College of Nursing.

Geden, E. et al. (1984). Self report and psychophysiological effects of five pain-coping strategies, *Nursing Research*, 33/5, 260–265.

Geissler, E.M. (1990). An exploratory study of selected female registered nurses: meaning and expression of nurturance, *Journal of Advanced Nursing*, 15, 5, 525–530.

Giorgi, A. (1971). An application of the phenomenological method in psychology, in Giorgi, A., Fisher, C. and Murray, E. (eds) *Duquesne Studies in Phenomenological Psychology* 2. Duquesne, Pittsburg University, 82–103.

Glaser, B., and Strauss, A. (1967). *The Discovery of Grounded Theory,* Chicago, Aldine.

Gold, R. (1958). Roles in sociological field observation, *Social Forces*, 36, 3, 217–223.

Gunter, L. (1981). Literature review, in Krampitz, S.B. and Pavlovich, M. (eds), *Readings for Nursing Research*, St. Louis, Mosby.

Hayes, R.J., Smith, P.G. and Carpenter, L. (1990). In letters to the editor, *The Lancet*, 336, 8724, 1185.

Hays, W.L. (1988). *Statistics.1988*, New York, Holt, Rinehart and Winston Inc.

Hedges, A. (1985). Group interviewing, in Walker, R. (eds) (1985). *Applied Qualitative Research,* Aldershot, Gower.

Heide, W.S. (1982).*Feminism for the Health of It*, Ann Arbor, Michigan, University Microfilms International.

Heidenreich, T. and Giuffre, M. (1990). Post-operative temperature measurement, *Nursing Research*, 39/3, 153–154.

Hendriksen, C. et al. (1984). Consequences of assessment and intervention among elderly people: a three year randomised controlled trial, *British Medical Journal*, 289, (1984), 1522–1525.

Hockey,E. (1987). Issues in the communication of nursing research, in Hockey, E. (ed),*Recent Advances in Nursing —Current Issues*, 1987, 18, Edinburgh, Churchill Livingstone.

Homans, G.C. (1958). Group factors in workers productivity, in Maccoby, E.E., Newcomb, T.M. and Hartley, E.L. (eds) *Readings in Social Psychology*, New York, Holt, Rinehart and Winston.

Howe, K.R. (1988). Against the quantitative – qualitative imcompatibility thesis, *Educational Researcher*, 17, 8, 10–16.

Hughes, C.C. (1992). Ethnography: what's in a word – process? product? promise?, *Qualitative Health Research*, 2, 4, 439–450.

Hughes, J.A. (1976). *Sociological Analysis: Methods of Discovery*, London, Nelson.

Husserl, E. (1965). *Phenomenology and the Crisis of Philosophy*, New York, Harper and Row.

Illich, I. (1977). *Limits to Medicine*, Harmondsworth, Penguin.

Jacob, E. (1987). Qualitative research traditions: a review, *Review of Educational Research*, 57, 1, 1–50.

Johnson, S.M. and Bolstad, B.D. (1973). Methodological issues in naturalistic observation: some problems and solutions for field research, in Hamerlynck, L.A. (ed), *Behaviour Change*, Champaign, Illinois, Research Press.

Jones, S. (1985). Depth interviewing, in Walker, R. (ed) (1985), *Applied Qualitative Research*, Aldershot, Gower.

Keller, C. (1991). Seeking normalcy: the experience of coronary artery bypass surgery, *Research in Nursing and Health*, 14, 173–178.

Kidder, L.H. (1981). *Seltiz, Wrightman and Cook's – Research Methods in Social Relations* (4th edition), London, Holt, Rinchart and Winston.

Kuhn, T.S. (1970). *The Structure of Scientific Revolutions*, Chicago, Chicago University Press.

Laudan, L. (1977). Progress and its problems: towards a scientific growth quoted in Munhall, P.L. and Oiler, C.J. (eds) (1986), *Nursing Research: A Qualitative Perspective*, Connecticut, Appleton Century Crofts.

Leininger, M. (1992). Current issues, problems and trends to advance qualitative paradigmatic research methods for the future, *Qualitative Health Research*, 2, 292–315.

Lincoln, Y. and Guba, E. (1985). *Naturalistic Enquiry*, Beverly Hills, C.A. Sage.

Lincoln, Y.S. (1992). Sympathetic connections between qualitative methods and health research, *Qualitative Health Research*, 2.4, 375–391.

Mead, G.H. (1934). *Mind, Self and Society,* Chicago, University of Chicago Press.

Mechanic, D. (1989). Medical sociology: some tensions among theory, method and substance, *Journal of Health and Social Behaviour,* 30, 147–160.

Merleau-Ponty, M. (1964). *The Primacy of Perception and other Essays on Phenomenological Psychology,* Evanston, Illinois, North Western University Press.

Milgram, S. (1963). Behavioural study of obedience, *Journal of Abnormal and Social Psychology,* 67, 371–374.

Milgram, S. (1964). Group pressure and action against a person, *Journal of Abnormal and Social Psychology,* 69, 137–143.

Millman, M. (1976).*The Unkindest Cut.,* New York, Morrow Quill.

Moreno, J. (1951). *Who Shall Survive? Foundations of Sociometry Group Psychotheropy and Sociodrama,* New York, Beacon House.

Munhall, P.L. and Oiler, C.J. (eds) (1986). *Nursing Research: A Qualitative Perspective,* Connecticut, Appleton Century Crofts.

National Health Service (NHS) – Management Executive(1991). *Research for Health: A Research and Development Strategy for the NHS,* London, NHS Management Executive.

Oiler, C. (1982). The phenomenological approach in nursing research. *Nursing Research,* 31(3), 178–181.

Orem, D.E. (1980). *Nursing: Concepts of Practice* (2nd Ed.), New York, McGraw Hill.

Parahoo, K. and Reid, N. (1988). Critical reading of research, *The Nursing Times,* 84, 43, 69–72.

Parahoo, K. and Reid, N. (1988). Research skills Number 4 – Writing up a research report, *Nursing Times,* 84, 42, 63–67.

Paterson, J. and Zderad, L. (1976). *Humanistic Nursing,* New York, Wiley.

Paykel, E.S. and Griffith, J.H. (1983). *Community Psychiatric Nursing for Neurotic Patients,* London, Royal College of Nursing.

Pirsig, R.M. (1974). *Zen and The Art of Motorcycle Maintenance,* London, Bodley Head.

Polanyi, M. (1958). *Personal Knowledge,*.Chicago, University of Chicago Press.

Popper, K.R. (1963). *Conjecture and Refutations, The Growth of Scientific Knowledge,* New York, Harper & Row.

Porter, S. (1991). A participant observation study of power relations between nurses and doctors in a general hospital, *Journal of Advanced Nursing*, 6, 728–735.

Posner, J. (1980). Urban anthropology: fieldwork in semi-familiar settings, in Shaffir, W.B. (ed.), *Fieldwork Experience*, New York, St. Martin's Press.

Reason, P. (1988). *Human Inquiry in Action, Developments in New Paradigm Research.*, London, Sage Publications.

Reason, P. and Rowan, J. (eds) (1981). *Human Inquiry: A Sourcebook of New Paradigm Research*, New York, John Wiley.

Reid, N. (1983). *A multivariate statistical investigation of the factors affecting nurse training in the clinical area*, Unpub, D.Phil. thesis, Coleraine, New University of Ulster.

Reinharz, S. (1981). Implementing new paradigm research, in Reason, P. and Rowan, J. (eds), *Human Inquiry: A Sourcebook of New Paradigm Research*, New York, John Wiley.

Ribbens, J. (1989). Interviewing – an 'unnatural situation'?, *Womeŋs Studies International Forum*, 12(6), 579–592.

Riehl, J.P. (1980). The Riehl Interaction Model, in Riehl, J.P. and Roy, C. (Ed), *Conceptual Models for Nursing Practice*. Norwalk, Appleton Century Crofts.

Robinson, J. (1990). Commenting on the 'Pink case' in *Nursing Standard*. 5, 7, 42.

Rogers, C. (1968). Some thoughts regarding the current presuppositions of the behavioral sciences, in Coulson, W. and Rogers, C. (eds) *Man and the Science of Man*, Columbus, Ohio, Charles E Merrill.

Rogers,C. (1985). Toward a more human science of the person, *J.of Humanistic Psychology*, 25,4,7–24.

Rosenhan, D.L. (1973). On being sane in insane places, *Science*, 179, 250–258.

Roy, C. (1980). The Roy adaptation model, in Riehl, J.P. and Roy. C. (ed) *Conceptual Models for Nursing Practice*, Norwalk, Appleton Century Crofts.

Ruffing-Rahal, M.A. (1991). Ethnographic traits in the writings of Mary Breckinridge, *Journal of Advanced Nursing*, 16, 614–620.

Sanders, C.R. (1980). Rope Burns: impediments to the achievement of comfort early in the field research experience, in Shaffir, W.B. (ed.), *Fieldwork Experience*, New York, St. Martin's Press.

Sartre, M. (1963). *Search for a Method*, New York, Vintage Books.

Schön, D. (1987). *Educating the Reflective Practitioner,* San Francisco, Jossey Bass.

Schutz. A, (1972). *The Phenomenology of the Social World,* London, Heinemann Educational Books.

Sellick, T. (1977). *Satisfying and anxiety creating incidents as identified by student nurses during the process of becoming a state registered nurse,* Unpub. MSc dissertation, Manchester, University of Manchester.

Siedman, E. (1977). Why not qualitative analysis, *Public Management Forum,* July/ August, 415–417.

Simmons, S. (1990). Family burden – what does psychiatric illness mean to the carers?, in Brooker, C. (ed) (1990), *Community Psychiatric Nursing: A Research Perspective,* London, Chapman and Hall.

Slevin, O.D'A. (1992). Knowledgeable doing: the theoretical basis for practice, in Slevin, O. and Buckenham, M. (eds), *Project 2000:The Teachers Speak,* Edinburgh, Campion Press.

Smith, C.E. et al. (1990). Diarrhea associated with tube feeding in mechanically ventilated critically ill patients, in *Nursing Research ,* 39/3 148–152.

Spiegelberg, H. (1976). *The Phenomenological Movement, Vol.I & II,* The Hague, Martinus Nifhoff.

Stewart, D. and Mickunas, A. (1974). *Exploring Phenomenology: A Guide to the Field and its Literature.* Chicago. American Library Association.

Strauss, A. and Corbin, J. (1990). *Basics of Qualitative Research,* London, Sage Publications.

United Kingdom Central Council for Nursing, Midwifery and Health Visiting (UKCC) (1986). *Project 2000: A New Preparation for Practice,* London, UKCC.

Van Kaam, A. (1959). Phenomenological analysis: exemplified in a study of the experience of being really understood, *Individual Psychology,* 15:66–72.

Verhonick, P.J. and Seaman, C.C. (1978). *Research Methods for Undergraduate Students of Nursing,* New York, Appleton Century Crofts.

Walker, L.O. (1989). A longitudinal analysis of stress problems among mothers of infants, in *Nursing Research* 38/6 339–343.

Walker, R. (eds) (1985). *Applied Qualitative Research,* Aldershot, Gower.

160

Webb, C. (1993). Feminist research: definitions, methodology, methods and evaluation, *J. of Advanced Nursing*, 18,416–423.

Webb, E.J., Campbell, B.T., Schwartz, R.D. and Sechrest, L. (1966). *Unobtrusive Measures*, Chicago, Rand McNally.

Weick, K.E. (1968). Systematic observational methods, in Lindsey, G. and Aronson, E. (eds), *The Handbook of Social Psychology*, Reading, Mass., Addison Wesley.

Wilkes, L. (1991). Phenomenology: a window to the nursing world, in Gray, A. and Pratt, R. (eds),*Towards a Discipline of Nursing*, London, Churchill Livingstone.

Wilkinson, S. (1986). *Feminist Social Psychology:Developing Theory and Practice*, Milton Keynes, Open University Press.

Wilson, J. (1989). Conceptual and empirical truth: some notes for researchers, *Educational Research*, 31, 3, 176–180.

INDEX